The Cold and Flu Cure

Dr. Susan's Healthy Living
drsusanshealthyliving.com

Facebook.com/DrSusanRichards
drsusanshealthyliving@gmail.com
(650) 561-9978

Mention of specific companies or products in this book does not suggest endorsement by the author or publisher. Internet addresses and telephone numbers for resources provided in this book were accurate at the time it went to press.

ISBN 978-1511958349

Note

The information in this book is meant to complement the advice and guidance of your physician, not replace it. It is very important that any person who has medical problems be evaluated by a physician. If you are under the care of a physician, you should discuss any major changes in your regimen with him or her. Because this is a book and not a medical consultation, keep in mind that the information presented here may not apply in your particular case. In view of individual medical requirements, new research, and government regulations, it is the responsibility of the reader to validate health practices and treatments with a physician or health service.

Table of Contents

Part I:
Understanding Respiratory Infections

1

There's Hope and Relief For You!

If you have been suffering from frequent colds, flus, sinusitis, middle ear infections or bronchitis, you don't need to look any further for help. I am so glad that you found this book! I wrote this book to share with you my truly ground breaking approach to successfully dealing with these energy sapping irritating nuisances that drain your energy and downgrade the quality of your life.

I developed my all natural program because so many of my patients were suffering from these common respiratory issues and they needed help. They needed solutions that really worked. The feedback from so many patients, friends and family over the years has been so positive that I felt that the millions of people suffering from these conditions needed access to this information.

First, I want to share with you one of my cases: my patient, Annie, whose colds and chronic bronchitis were so severe and so frequent that they drastically affected the quality of her life and even her ability to work.

When I first started to work with Annie, she was very sickly. During our first visit, she was constantly coughing, blowing her nose, and sneezing. She complained of chest tightness and, at times, even seemed to be gasping for breath.

Of even greater concern was that her respiratory issues seemed to be getting worse. Her symptoms were now recurring every few weeks, particularly during times of stress. All of her stress seemed to go into her lungs and trigger respiratory infections. She worked as a consultant so she depended on being able to meet regularly with her clients. As her health worsened, she was finding that she was cancelling appointments more and more frequently.

At our initial office visit, she shared with me that she had recently experienced some extreme upset and discord with her family and was so upset that she had developed a severe episode of bronchitis and couldn't work for nearly a week. Annie felt tired constantly and had very low energy. She knew that she should exercise regularly but felt too tired to make the effort.

When I took her medical history, it was obvious to me that her stress and lack of exercise, her nutritional deficiencies and overly acidic diet were contributing to her impaired respiratory health and the poor ventilation of her lungs, which were a breeding ground for unhealthy microorganisms.

I started her on a program of all natural, safe and effective alkalinizing substances, antimicrobials, enzymes, and other anti-inflammatory therapies as well as on a diet supportive of her respiratory health.

Annie was very motivated to become stronger. Fed up with feeling so weak and tired from her poor respiratory function, she took a breathing class and spent an evening learning exercises to support her lung function. (I share some great breathing exercises with you in this book.)

As her respiratory infections became less frequent and her immunity strengthened, she began to swim at least four days a week and began an early morning stretching class once a week.

After suffering from years of respiratory infections and weakness, Annie rarely becomes sick with colds and bronchitis anymore. When she is under more stress and starts to cough, she just increases her maintenance program and steps up her protective supplements and her symptoms disappear without ever developing into an infection.

There is now a sparkle in her eye and her face looks brighter and more alive. She is very excited about her stronger immunity and rarely misses appointments with her clients now.

Many of my patients not only want to be free of respiratory infections for themselves, but also are equally concerned about their children, given the prevalence of colds, flus, middle ear infections, and sinus and chest congestion.

I also want to share with you the story my patient, Jessica, and her daughter Sarah. When Sarah was an infant and small child up to the age of eighteen months, she was plagued with constant ear infections and colds. Sarah was adopted at four months so she was only formula fed and didn't received the immune supportive benefits of breastfeeding. In addition, her pediatrician kept prescribing antibiotics that probably threw her further out of balance since it killed off her normal healthy flora as well as the disease causing bacteria. This probably contributed to her digestive issues included frequent diarrhea that concerned Jessica greatly.

Jessica and I discussed these issues, I recommended that she begin Sarah on probiotics to replenish her healthy, normal flora as well as digestive enzymes, and bovine colostrum. Sarah responded immediately and her colds and ear infections began to diminish. By the age of two, Jessica added a high quality multi-nutrient product and omega 3 fatty acids, which are potent anti-inflammatories to Sarah's program. Sarah is now five years old and is a strong, healthy and very active little girl. She rarely gets colds and has never had an ear infection again since beginning my program.

You and your family can enjoy the same amazing recovery and health benefits as Jessica and Sarah with my program. There are five steps to this program that will make you virtually invincible to colds, flus and lung infections. They will give you a shield of protection so that respiratory infections rarely develop, and if one does, you will be able to recover from it much more rapidly than ever before. I share all of these steps with you in my book.

The five steps include destroying respiratory causing pathogens through the use of safe, all natural antimicrobial agents; healthy detoxification and the destruction of viruses, bacteria and toxins; the ability to suppress inflammation through the use of pancreatic and plant enzymes and other anti-inflammatory substances; healthy buffering capacity (restoring a slightly alkaline pH to your cells and tissues); and the ability to keep our cells and tissues well oxygenated.

My program can greatly benefit people of all ages from adults, children, and even infants. However, the dosages of the treatments will often vary depending on age. I have included the appropriate dosages for infants, children, and adults in my book. Teenagers and adults can usually take the regular dosages mentioned in this book; children and infants need much smaller dosages.

As with adults, I have found that children do extremely well with my program. It has been very exciting to me to see ailing children who are constantly plagued with respiratory infections become strong and healthy. With my program you and your children can become free from the uncomfortable symptoms of colds, flus, middle ear infections, and sinus and chest congestion and have these issues disappear from your life.

If you have specific questions and concerns about giving your child nutritional supplements, it is best to check with your own health care provider.

Pregnant and nursing woman are in a special category of their own. They should only take supplements with the approval of their health care provider.

I will discuss each of these five steps in detail in this book. By following my program, you will be well on your way to saying good-bye to colds, flus, sinusitis, middle ear infections, and bronchitis forever!

Respiratory Infections Are Among Our Most Common Illnesses

Like Annie, millions of people in our country struggle with respiratory infections on an ongoing basis. The statistics on the prevalence of respiratory ailments reflect how common these conditions are in the United States. There are over one billion cases of the common cold annually that result in either medical treatment or at least one day of restricted activity. This is an astounding figure, but not too surprising since many children and adults suffer from as many as four to six colds each year.

In addition, there are nearly 37 million cases of chronic sinusitis, 14 million cases of chronic bronchitis, and 14.5 million cases of asthma annually.

Millions of children and adults also suffer flu-like illness as well as from middle ear infections and bronchitis each year. The prevalence of respiratory infections translates into an enormous drain on both individual and corporate resources as well as huge outlays of money spent on treating these conditions.

To counteract these ailments, Americans spend billions of dollars on over-the-counter remedies. In fact, in 2008, cold, cough, and sore throat sufferers spent over $4.6 billion dollars on remedies for these conditions.

Unfortunately, these over-the-counter products are relatively ineffective and have unpleasant, and even serious, side effects. They only provide partial symptom relief and do not help to restore the health and balance of the body that is needed to recover rapidly from these conditions.

Quality of life, and even the ability to just show up at work or social engagements, can be hampered by common respiratory illnesses. The symptoms that accompany these conditions can seriously interfere with a person's ability to fulfill their job, household, and family responsibilities, much less perform at optimal levels.

Additionally, colds and flus are one of the most common reasons for children to miss school; and constant absenteeism due to these conditions can greatly affect a child's ability to learn and keep up with the rest of the class.

All of these conditions drastically reduce people's energy, create sleep disturbances, and impair concentration. They also greatly hamper socializing and make travel unpleasant. Their symptoms often occur at inopportune times and hinder consistent performance, causing them to make uncharacteristic mistakes on the job. In addition, individuals with minor illnesses often feel miserable and tend to isolate themselves from coworkers, friends, and family members.

In my clinical practice, I often see people who have had acute sinus conditions, colds, flus, and bronchial infections that have taken anywhere from one to six weeks to be completely resolved, despite the use of prescription or over-the-counter drugs, which often simply substitute one set of lingering symptoms for another and do not cure the underlying causes. These conditions are truly major hindrances in enjoying and participating in one's daily life.

Medications Don't Cure Respiratory Infections

Unfortunately, there are no cures for the common cold or for most respiratory infections. The medications used mostly provide only symptom relief and often create uncomfortable side effects that can negate their benefits.

The medications themselves often increase conditions like over acidity, which is the perfect environment for cold and flu causing microbes to thrive, often retriggering the symptoms. No matter what medications respiratory illness sufferers use, recovery can be prolonged if the underlying over acidity and other imbalances of the system are not corrected.

Besides medications, physicians usually just recommend rest, eating lightly and a few self-care therapies like gargling with saltwater or using a humidifier.

I will discuss the different medications and their side effects later on in this book so that you are fully informed about their effects on the body.

Natural Therapies Can Greatly Decrease Respiratory Infections

Happily, I have found that both the frequency and symptoms of respiratory infections can be greatly reduced through the use of safe, all natural therapies. In fact, the benefits of my program are so dramatic that even people who suffer from repeated respiretory infections can gain significant relief so that these infections become very rare and, often, disappear entirely.

In Part I of this book, I provide a strong foundation of information for you so that you can better understand these conditions. I share important facts about respiratory infections as well as discussing their symptoms, diagnosis and conventional treatment. I also discuss the drugs commonly used to treat these infections and their side effects and drawbacks.

In Part II, I discuss the five essential therapies that, when used together, offer dramatic relief from and prevention of respiratory infections. I give you detailed information about these therapies and how best to work with them along with important recovery tips.

By following my program, you will be well on your way towards saying good-bye to colds, flus, sinusitis, middle ear infections, and bronchitis forever!

Let's get started!

2

Facts About and The Symptoms of Respiratory Infections

First, I want to discuss important facts about and the symptoms of the most common types of respiratory infections. I have included checklists of the symptoms to help you assess the severity of your own condition. The diagnosis of many common respiratory conditions, like colds and flus, are primarily made by assessing the symptoms and by physical examination. Physicians often do not run laboratory tests unless they are indicated.

Common Colds

Common colds are caused by viral infections of the upper respiratory tract. This includes the nose, sinuses, Eustachian tubes, throat, trachea, larynx and bronchial tubes. Over 200 different viruses have been identified as causing colds, but the most common groups are rhinoviruses and coronaviruses.

While preschool and grade school children catch colds most frequently, adolescents and adults develop colds, too. Children often catch colds from their classmates in school or daycare centers. Parents can catch colds from their infected children. It is not unusual to see colds spread through entire families. While colds can occur during any time of the year, they are most common during the autumn, winter and early spring, the colder and rainy months of the year.

As mentioned earlier, there are over one billion colds each year in the United States. Many people suffer from at least several colds per year. Colds are the most common cause of children missing school and adults missing work.

Once you are infected, the cold virus attaches itself to the mucosal lining of the sinuses or nasal passages. In response, the infected tissues begin to release a chemical called histamine. This chemical increases the blood flow and inflammation to the infected area, causing increased mucous production, swelling and congestion. Within one to three days, the typical symptoms of colds begin to appear.

If you have a cold, you are contagious during the first two to three days after the onset of symptoms. You can be infected through contact with another person when you breathe in little virus containing fluid droplets that are expelled on coughing, sneezing, blowing the nose or speaking.

Colds may also be passed by direct contact if you touch your nose, mouth or eyes after touching either an infected person or infected object like a doorknob or toy.

Colds are usually diagnosed through the person's symptoms and medical history. Laboratory testing is rarely done unless your doctor suspects a secondary infection.Since colds are caused by viruses, they should not be treated with antibiotics. Medications offering symptom relief are usually recommended by physicians. However, many of these medications cause side-effects and they do not cure the common cold.

Colds Self Quiz

The most common symptoms of colds are listed in this self quiz. Read through this list to see which ones apply to you or a family member.

- nasal congestion, stuffy nose
- runny nose
- postnasal drip
- sneezing
- watery eyes
- sore or scratchy throat
- low grade fever (in children) of no more than 100-102 degrees F.
- cough
- chills
- headache
- decreased appetite
- muscle aches

For most people, these symptoms begin to subside within a week or ten days. But people with decreased immunity the symptoms can linger for several weeks or even a month. Colds also make you more susceptible to secondary infections like middle ear infections, bronchitis, or sinusitis.

Influenza

Influenza, commonly called the flu, is an infectious disease caused by RNA viruses of the family Orthomyxoviridae (the influenza virus). These viruses commonly affect birds and mammals.

Influenza tends to spread throughout the world in seasonal epidemics. Pandemics of influenza occurred in the 20th century, killing million of people. New strains of influenza virus tend to occur frequently which can make treatment and containment of the epidemics more difficult with each new epidemic. These epidemics can be quite contagious. Approximately 41,000 people died each year from influenza in the United States between 1979-2001.

The flu virus is typically transmitted as an airborne infection, through sneezes and coughs expelling air borne droplets that contain the virus. It can also be transmitted by direct contact through nasal secretions, contact with contaminated surfaces and objects and even bird droppings. Luckily, the virus can be inactivated by soap, disinfectant and even sunlight. As a result, frequent hand washing and the use of sanitary hand wipes can confer some protection and reduce the risk of infection, especially if you are in contact with a person who is already is ill.

Initially, the symptoms may seem similar to those of a common cold with nasal congestion, sore throat, sneezing, dry cough and achiness. However, the flu symptoms come on much more suddenly than those of a cold and are more severe. Fever is often higher than that seen with a cold. The temperature can rise as high as 100 to 104 degrees F, and even as high as 106 degrees when symptoms first occur. Fever is often worse in children and teenagers than adults and often begins to go down after a few days.

One of the biggest concerns with the flu is the development of pneumonias, a secondary infection. Pneumonia can either be due to viral infection, or even a bacterial pneumonia, which can be very dangerous if not treated immediately.

If a person with the flu seems to be getting better and then relapses with a high fever or begins to have trouble breathing, you should suspect pneumonia and seek immediate medical care. Doctors may choose to treat the patient with both antibiotics and anti-viral medication. Physicians often recommend the flu vaccine to individuals who are at risk like the elderly.

Influenza is usually diagnosed without laboratory testing, especially if it occurs during the flu season. Testing may be prescribed, however, by physicians in times of severe epidemics to help recognize the infections early and minimize their spread, especially in compromised patients or those at higher risk.

Influenza Self Quiz

The most common symptoms of influenza are listed in this self quiz. Read through this list to see which ones apply to you or a family member.

- fever over 100 degrees F
- muscle aches in the throat, back, arms and legs
- sore throat
- chills, shivering and sweating
- dry cough
- nasal congestion
- headache
- fatigue and weakness
- watery, irritated eyes
- diarrhea and abdominal pain in children
- pneumonia, in severe cases

Sinusitis

The sinuses are air-filled spaces in the skull that are lined with mucous membranes. They are located in the areas of the eyes, cheeks, nasal bones and forehead. When the function of these sinuses is healthy, mucous production is minimal and the mucous formed can readily drain our. Air is also able to circulate within these spaces.

Sinusitis can occur when too much mucous is produced or the sinus openings become blocked. This can frequently occur due to colds and allergies; when small hairs in the sinuses called cilia do not function properly; or if the person has nasal polyps or a deviated nasal septum that can block the opening of the sinuses.

Acute sinusitis is usually caused by a bacterial or viral infection and develops rapidly. This type of sinusitis usually clears up in less than four weeks. It often follows a cold that does not improve or becomes worse after five to seven days.

In contrast, chronic sinusitis normally lasts three months or longer and is often caused by a bacterial or fungal infection. While symptoms may sometimes be milder, chronic sinusitis can cause damage in the mucous membranes that line the sinuses.

To diagnose sinusitis, your physician will take your medical history and look inside the nose for mucous or pus draining from the sinuses or signs of polyps. Physicians may use a small, thin telescope-like device called an endoscope to do this. They may also shine a light into your nasal passages in order to see inflammation or fluid.

Your physician may also take nasal and sinus cultures of the mucous discharge to determine if you have a bacterial or fungal infection. This is usually done if your symptoms are not resolving rapidly. Physicians may request a CT (computerized tomography) scan that can visualize physical obstruction or deep pockets of inflammation. The CT scan can visualize soft tissue and other structures that can't be seen on a regular x-ray.

Antibiotics are usually not prescribed for acute sinusitis since these infections tend to clear up on their own. However, your physician may suspect a bacterial infection and prescribe antibiotics if your nasal discharge contains pus, gets worse after five days or persists for several weeks. Antibiotics may also be prescribed if you have a child with these symptoms who is not getting better after several weeks.

Sinusitis Self Quiz

The most common symptoms of sinusitis are listed in this self-quiz. Read through this list to see which ones apply to you or a family member.

- thick yellow or greenish discharge from the nose or down the back of the throat
- nasal congestion
- difficulty breathing through the nose
- facial pain and swelling, especially around your nose, cheeks, eyes, ears or forehead
- aching sensation in the teeth or upper jaw
- diminished sense of taste or smell
- cough
- sore throat
- bad breath
- fatigue and tiredness

Middle Ear Infections (Otitis Media)

Ear infections are among the most common reasons for medical visits to the doctor for children. The most common type of ear infection is called otitis media that refers to infection and inflammation of the middle ear.

The middle ear is the area behind the eardrum (or tympanic membrane) and the inner ear. It also includes a structure called the Eustachian tube, which runs from the middle ear to the back of the throat. This tube helps to drain fluid normally made in the middle ear.

The Eustachian tubes can easily become blocked and swollen from colds, sinusitis, allergies, teething in infants and even environmental pollutants like cigarette smoke. When these tubes are blocked, the fluid in the middle ear can accumulate and infection can occur. This is very commonly seen in infants and children. It can also occur in adults, though less frequently.

Ear infections are seen more commonly during the winter months, but can occur any time of the year if a child or adult is predisposed to developing them. These infections can be caused either by a virus or bacteria.

While earache or ear pain are the most common symptoms in adults and older children, in infants the main symptoms may be constant crying and irritability as well as difficulty sleeping. Since all middle ear infections involve fluid build up behind the eardrum, drainage of fluid from the ear may be a sign of a ruptured eardrum.

To diagnose middle ear infection, your health care provider will look inside the ears with an instrument called an otoscope that allows you to look at the ear canal and the eardrum itself. With a middle ear infection, the eardrum may be red and inflamed looking. There may be bloody fluid or pus as well as a hole or perforation of the eardrum.

The treatments recommended by physicians are primarily for symptom relief including the use of over the counter medications for pain such as ibuprofen or acetaminophen and pain relief drops. However, your health care provider may prescribe antibiotics if the patient is not improving within 24 to 48 hours, has a fever or if your child is under the age of two.

Middle Ear Infections Self Quiz

The most common symptoms of sinusitis are listed in this self quiz. Read through this list to see which ones apply to you or a family member.

Children

- ear pain or earache, worse on lying down
- drainage of fluid from the ear
- pulling at ear
- difficulty sleeping
- irritability
- diminished hearing in the affected ear
- headache
- fever of 100 degrees F or higher
- loss of appetite, nausea, vomiting, diarrhea

Adults

- ear pain or earache
- drainage of fluid from the ear
- loss of hearing in the affected ear
- sore throat

Bronchitis

Bronchitis occurs when there is inflammation of the main air passages to the lungs that causes a persistent cough. Acute bronchitis is a shorter terms condition that usually occurs following a viral respiratory infection.

Symptoms first affect the sinuses, nose and throat and then can spread to the lungs. Occasionally, bacteria can infect the lungs along with the viral infection, causing a secondary bacterial infection that then must be treated with antibiotics in addition to medications for symptom relief that are usually recommended by physicians. I discuss these medications and their side-effects later on in the book.

Symptoms of acute bronchitis usually clear up within seven to ten days; however the cough can linger for weeks. You are at higher risk of acute bronchitis if you have preexisting heart or lung disease. The elderly, young children, and smokers are also at higher risk.

Some people suffer from chronic bronchitis, which is a longer-term condition. A chronic persistent cough with mucous production and difficulty breathing are typically seen with this condition. It is often seen in smokers and is considered to be one type of chronic obstructive pulmonary disease (COPD).

Physicians often prescribe inhalers (bronchodilators) to open up the airways as well as inhaled steroids to suppress lung inflammation. Oxygen therapy may be needed in severe cases.

Your health care provider will usually listen to your lungs with a stethoscope to see if there are sounds called rales or other abnormal breathing sounds. Your physician may also order a chest x-ray or CT scan as well as take a sputum sample to check for bacterial infection.

If you have chronic bronchitis, your physician may order lung function tests or check the level of oxygen in your blood.

Pneumonia can develop as a complication from both acute and chronic bronchitis. This serious condition must be diagnosed and aggressively treated when it occurs.

Bronchitis Self Quiz

The most common symptoms of bronchitis are listed in this self-quiz. Read through this list to see which ones apply to you or a family member.

- persistent cough, dry or mucous producing
- yellow or green mucous production, may be streaked with blood
- fever below 101 degrees F (a higher fever may indicate pneumonia)
- chills
- tightness, pain or burning sensation in the chest
- pain below breastbone with deep breathing
- shortness of breath
- wheezing or hoarseness

3

The Problems with Medications

For many of us, the usual response to the onset of colds, flus and lung infections is to run to the pharmacy to try to find products that will give relief to the uncomfortable symptoms. Often, your own doctor will suggest these therapies because prescription drugs are rarely appropriate for the treatment of respiratory infections.

Your doctor will normally only prescribe medication if your condition has been proven to be due to a bacterial or fungal infection or is serious enough to requite prescription anti-inflammatory drugs for chronic bronchitis. Prescription antiviral agents may also be used in the early stages of influenza if you are at risk of complications.

Unfortunately, there are significant problems with using over the counter medications for respiratory conditions. These medications do not cure the problem or shorten its duration but only offer some symptom relief. Even worse, they often cause side effects that may be more uncomfortable and debilitating than the respiratory infection itself! If used for more than a few days, your symptoms may actually worsen with some of the OTC medications. In addition, these medications should never be used in children under the age of two and these products haven't been shown to be safe or effective for children under the age of six.

Let's look at some of the common OTC medications used to treat respiratory infections.

Antihistamines are taken to relieve symptoms such as nasal congestion, runny nose, sneezing, watery eyes and itching of the eyes. These drugs include Chlor-Trimeton, Dimetapp, and Actifed (which contain an antihistamine and decongestant). Side effects of these medications include drowsiness, sleepiness, dizziness, dry mouth, nausea, vomiting, constipation and, in severe cases, difficulty urinating, confusion, hallucinations, and visual problems like blurred or double vision. Any of these serious side effects should be reported to your doctor.

Decongestants are taken to relieve nasal congestion, sinus congestion and open inflamed, swollen nasal passages, thereby making breathing easier. They also are used to reduce inflammation in the throat by constricting blood vessels in this area. They are also used in nasal sprays and eye drops. They create this effect within the body by enhancing the activity of excitatory chemicals like norepinephrine (noradrenaline) and epinephrine (adrenaline).

Decongestants are available in pill form that can be taken orally. These include Sudafed 12 Hour (pseudoephedrine) and Sudafed PE (phenylephrine). They are also available over the counter as nasal sprays and drops.

Unfortunately, the effects of these drugs aren't limited to just the respiratory tract. They often cause very uncomfortable side effects and are not well tolerated by many people. Side effects including nervousness, anxiety, sleeplessness, dizziness, over excitability, rapid heart rate, increased blood pressure, urinary problems, and visual changes.

Overuse of decongestant nasal sprays and drops for longer than three days can even cause a rebound effect causing the blood vessels in the nose to swell thereby making your nasal congestion even worse.

Antitussives are commonly used in cough medications. Many over the counter medications such as Benylin and Benylin DM contain antitussives like dextromethorphan. Dextromethorphan works by decreasing activity in the brain that causes coughing. Side effects include rashes, drowsiness, itching, nausea, dizziness and difficulty breathing. Its use should be avoided in individuals with a known history of allergic reactions. Eating grapefruit or drinking grapefruit juice should be avoided when using dextromethorphan containing medication since it can affect the metabolism of this substance.

Expectorants like guaifenesin helps to thin out and loosen mucous in your chest and throat. This allows excess mucous to be coughed up more easily so that the bronchial passages are cleared. Medications containing gauifenesin include Alifen, Mucinex, and Hytuss. Side effects can include allergic reactions such as hives, swelling of the face, lips, tongue or throat and difficulty breathing. Other side effects include dizziness, headache, rashes, nausea and vomiting.

Ache and Pain Relievers are often used for the relief of symptoms like muscle aches, generalized achiness, headaches and fever that accompany colds, flus and other respiratory infections. Commonly prescribed drugs include Tylenol (acetaminophen) that works by elevation of the pain threshold within the brain. Another type of medication used to relieve aches and pain are NSAIDs (nonsteroidal anti-inflammatory drugs). These types of drugs include aspirin and ibuprofen (Advil, Motrin). NSAIDs reduce pain by decreasing the production of prostaglandins. These are hormone-like substances that we produce within our bodies that can cause pain and inflammation.

Side effects of Tylenol include allergic reactions such as rashes, hives, difficulty breathing, tightness of the chest and swelling of the lips, tongue, or face. Other adverse effects include liver and kidney damage, nausea and vomiting, changes in blood pressure, headaches, muscle spasms, insomnia, anxiety, and fatigue.

NSAIDs cause equally worrisome side effects. These include nausea, vomiting, diarrhea, constipation, ulcers and gastrointestinal bleeding, drowsiness, rashes, headaches, dizziness, decreased appetite, and, most seriously, kidney and liver failure.

Some companies try to compound the benefits and unfortunately, the potential for side effects, by combining many of these categories so that antihistamines, decongestants, pain medication and a cough suppressant are all found in the same medication. Examples of these combination medications include Tylenol Cold, Sudafed Plus, Triaminic, and Tavist D.

As a general rule, it is best to avoid these medications and their potential for significant side effects. There are many other supportive steps that can be taken to improve the level of comfort while recovering from a respiratory infection that I will describe next.

Antibiotics are incredibly helpful medications when used properly, but disease resistance has occurred over the years because they have been overprescribed.

As a result they need to be prescribed carefully and only when absolutely indicated.

Yet, even antibiotics, which are appropriate and indicated for severe respiratory bacterial infections, have their downsides since they often cause side effects of their own. Since antibiotics are usually not needed for the treatment of respiratory infections which are often caused by viruses.

Antibiotics kill the normal, healthy bacteria that inhabit our intestinal tract. This can change the flora in our intestines and affect out ability to absorb essential nutrients like vitamins and minerals. It can also result in the overgrowth of yeast and cause diarrhea and digestive upset as well as more serious side effects. Overuse of antibiotics can also result in future infections developing from more serious and drug resistant organisms.

Rather than using medications that provide only partial symptom relief and often produce significant side effects, there is a better way. My program will help you to banish respiratory infections forever by eliminating both the causes and internal conditions that breed these infections. I share the details of this program with you in Part II of this book.

Supportive Therapies that Make You More Comfortable

While the following supportive measures do not cure respiratory infections or shorten the course of the illness, they can help you feel more comfortable and reduce the severity of the symptoms while you are recovering.

Eat Lightly While Recovering: It is important to eat lightly when recovering from colds, flus, and lung infections. It is also important to avoid acidic foods and beverages (more about this in the next section). Traditional home remedies for colds and flus include drinking a glass of orange juice or ginger ale to settle the stomach, or eating a bowl of Jell-O. While these might seem like comfort foods, they are highly acidic and will actually prolong recovery time.

Instead, you should drink herbal teas (ginger tea is particularly good for the treatment of colds and flus) or vegetable or chicken broths. A team of researchers at the University of Nebraska Medical Center published their findings in the journal *Chest*.

Most importantly, they found that chicken soup has an anti-inflammatory effect since chicken soup helped to stop the movement of neutrophils. These are while blood cells that engulf bacteria and cellular debris and are released in large numbers with viral infections like colds. Neutrophil activity can trigger the release of mucous that is a major symptom of colds and other respiratory infections. Either home-made or canned chicken soup will work!

For the first twelve to twenty-four hours after the onset of symptoms, taking in plenty of therapeutic teas and soups and avoiding solid food will help to bring the pH back into balance more rapidly.

Drink Plenty of Fluids: Be sure to drink plenty of water along with teas, broths, and soups. This will help to loosen mucous and prevent dehydration. This is particularly important if you have a fever.

Saltwater Gargles: A saltwater gargle, made with ¼ to ½ teaspoon of salt dissolved in a glass of warm water can provide temporary relief of scratchy and sore throats.

Saline Nasal Drops and Sprays: These saline-based products are far safer than the usual nasal decongest-ants found in your local pharmacy since they don't cause a rebound effect. The rebound effect is caused by overuse of decongestant drugs that actually make nasal swelling and congestion worse.

Nasal saline irrigation can also be done with a neti pot to flush the sinuses, reduce congestion and facial pain and pressure. However, it is important to be aware that several individuals were recently reported to have developed brain infections from the use of a neti pot. As a result, you may want to use the other options for saline irrigation, instead.

Apply Moisture to Your Face, Sinuses and Airway Passages. You can do this by applying a warm, moist washcloth to your face several times a day to reduce congestion in your sinuses and nasal passageways or over your ear if you have an earache. Humidifiers and steam inhalers can be useful for colds, flus, sinus infections and bronchial infections by relieving congestion, soothing sore throats and opening up air passageways to support more comfortable breathing.

Get Plenty of Rest While Recovering. It is very beneficial while recovering from a respiratory infection to reduce your work and activity schedule and spend more time resting. This will help to take extra stress off of your immune system so that your energy can be used for healing.

Avoid Changes in Your Environment. If at all possible, avoid flying when you are congested since the altitude changes and the closed in cabin can impede recovery. In addition, avoid temperature extremes or sudden changes in temperature.

Part II:
My Program-The Better Way to Heal from Respiratory Infections

4

Summary of Program

In Part II of my book, I will share with you five types of therapies that, when used together, offer dramatic relief from respiratory infections. My program will also help to prevent the recurrence of respiratory infections so that they become less and less frequent in your life.

These include: the use of powerful, natural antimicrobials to suppress the bacteria and viruses that cause these infections; healthy buffering capability (the ability to alkalinize your cells and tissues); the ability to suppress inflammation through the production of pancreatic enzymes and other anti-inflammatory substances, healthy detoxification, and the ability to keep our cells and tissues well oxygenated.

By following this program, you will be well on your way towards saying good-bye to colds, flus, sinusitis, middle ear infections, and bronchitis forever!

5

Antimicrobials

Since colds, flus, and lung infections are caused by pathogens like bacteria, viruses, and fungi, the first line of treatment is to destroy these disease causing organisms. This will help to speed up recovery by taking stress off of the immune system and reducing the severity of the symptoms.

In conventional medicine, antibiotics are used only for serious bacterial infections. Otherwise, the treatment for most respiratory infections is symptomatic. Happily, there are a number of powerful, safe, all natural therapies that either destroy microbes or boost and strengthen immunity. I discuss a number of them in this chapter.

Colloidal Silver

Colloidal silver is one of my favorite antimicrobial agents. I have seen numerous patients with respireatory infections benefit from its use. For centuries, silver has been known to be an effective antibacterial substance. In ancient civilizations, water was stored in silver vessels to keep bacteria from growing in it, and people in the nineteenth century often put a silver dollar in milk to retard spoilage. In the early twentieth century, colloidal silver was shown to be a very effective antibiotic and antiviral substance for eliminating or preventing many minor internal and external infections. Today it is recognized that colloidal silver is effective against over 650 disease-causing organisms.

I have found colloidal silver to be very effective in helping to combat colds, flus and lung conditions like bronchitis, shortening the course of the illnesses and helping to reduce symptoms. It is readily available in health food stores or for purchase on the Internet.

A colloid is a substance that consists of extremely fine particles suspended in another medium such as water. Colloidal silver is, therefore, submicroscopic clusters of pure metallic silver suspended in distilled water. It is created by electrolysis: An electrical current is passed between two poles, one of which is pure silver. The electric current breaks off micro-scopic pieces of the silver (a particle size of 0.0001 micron), and these particles stay suspended in the water due to their electrical charge. The particles are measured in parts per million (ppm); most products commercially available range from 5 to 500 ppm.

Studies show that many viruses, bacteria, and fungi are rendered ineffective (in vitro) in three to four minutes after exposure to colloidal silver. Although the exact mechanism of action is not known, it appears that the silver affects enzymes in the cells of the bacteria, inhibiting their replication.

Colloidal silver is nontoxic at prescribed doses. It is tasteless and odorless and can be taken orally or applied to the skin by either spraying it on or using it in a salve form. It does not irritate the eyes, and when applied to wounds or scrapes, it does not sting. Even though it is a powerful antibiotic, when taken in prescribed doses, it does not destroy the "friendly" bacteria in the intestinal tract. Unlike pharmaceutical antibiotics, colloidal silver never permits strain-resistant pathogens to develop. Colloidal silver can be used wherever and whenever an antibacterial or antiviral agent is indicated. It can be used both to treat existing conditions and as a preventive agent.

Colloidal silver can be purchased at health food stores. It is available in dropper bottles in strengths varying from 5 to 500 ppm. (Lower strengths of 5 to 10 ppm are probably optimal). When taking it orally, you should allow it to remain in the mouth for thirty to sixty seconds so that the microscopic particles of pure silver can be absorbed through the mucosal lining, bypassing the digestive tract. When using it on the skin, transfer the colloidal silver solution to a spray bottle and spray it on the affected area.

My patient, Veronica, shared a story with me in which colloidal silver helped to save her vacation.

She and her husband, Mike, took a trip to the Napa Valley, the beautiful wine country of California, for a weekend get away in the early spring. They were enjoying wine tasting along with the beautiful scenery when she began to come down with a violent cold. She began to have bouts of sneezing, and coughing and a great deal of nasal congestion.

Since she tends to suffer from colds, she had brought a bottle of colloidal silver with her along with enzymes and sodium bicarbonate, a program that I had shared with her when she originally came to see me as a patient. She started to take the colloidal silver and the other supplements every few hour. Her symptoms began to diminish very quickly and she was able to enjoy the rest of her holiday.

Suggested Dosage: Take two dropperfuls every two to four hours for an acute respiratory infection. Decrease to every six to eight hours as symptoms begin to resolve or after day 1 of treatment. For children, use one quarter to one half teaspoon two to three times a day. For children under five, give two drops of colloidal silver per pound of body weight. While the short-term use of colloidal silver is very safe, consult your health care practitioner if you have any questions about the use of colloidal silver with your child.

Hold dosage under the tongue for several minutes. Take colloidal silver on an empty stomach. Do not use colloidal silver on a long-term basis as it can cause a greyish discoloration of the skin called argyria.

My favorite product is Silver Biotics. It can be ordered through 801-756-1000 or Amazon.com.

Probiotics (Lactobacilli and Bifidobacetria)

Friendly bacteria like lactobacilli and bifidobacteria normally colonize the intestinal tract. These bacteria have many beneficial effects on digestion. Because they aid in the production of essential B vitamins as well as acetic and lactic acids, they prevent colonization of the colon by harmful bacteria and yeast.

Research studies have shown probiotic therapy to be useful for a number of health conditions, including respiratory infections. Certain strains of probiotics have also been shown to be helpful for vaginal and urinary tract infections, irritable bowel syndrome, ulcerative colitis and Crohn's disease.

Probiotic therapy has also been found to be very useful for the treatment of diarrhea in children. Research studies have shown that Lactobacillus GG can shorten the length of infectious diarrhea in children and even infants.

Unfortunately, the overconsumption of alcohol or sugar and a high-fat diet can reduce the population of beneficial lactobacilli and predispose the body to an overgrowth of harmful bacteria and fungi. Pathogenic organisms like candida may flourish in this environment.

I have also worked with numerous patients who have been given antibiotics to treat respiratory illnesses such as bronchitis and the flu and have consequently developed candida. The vaginal itching, burning, and discharge due to overgrowth of candida in the vagina and intestines then has to be treated as a separate infection.

A number of research studies have shown the benefits of probiotics supplementation for children with respiratory infections. In the *Supplement to Pediatrics*, a research study reported that children between the ages of 6 to 12 months were either given specific strains of Lactobacillus Acidophilus, a combination of Lactobacillus Acidophilus and Bifidobacterium Lactis, or a placebo. The probiotics were ingested daily for six months, from November to April. These are peak months for respiratory infections.

Symptoms such as fever, cough, and nasal congestion were significantly reduced in both probiotic treatment groups compared to the children who only received the placebo. The benefits were especially strong in the group of children taking the combination probiotic therapy. In addition, children in the placebo group had, on average, 6.5 days of symptoms while those in the Lactobacillus Acidophilus group had 4.5 days of symptoms and in the combination treatment group they had only 3.4 days of symptoms. These are dramatic benefits from the use of probiotics in children!

In another study, both Lactobacillus rhamnosus GG and Bifidobacterium Lactis strains were given daily to infants in their formula and were found to significantly reduce the risk of acute middle-ear infection during the first year of life compared to the infants given placebo.

A seven month, double-blind, placebo-controlled study of 571 children in day care centers in Finland were treated with milk fortified with the probiotic Lactobacillus GG. The treatment did reduce the frequency and severity of respiratory infections.

Research studies have also found probiotics to be effective in reducing the frequency of respiratory symptoms and their severity in adults, too. In one controlled study reported in the *British Journal of Sports Medicine*, endurance athletes, specifically long distance runners, were treated with probiotics for four months. Probiotic therapy helped to protect these athletes from respiratory infections. Intensive exercise can suppress healthy immune function and make athletes more vulnerable to respiratory infections such as colds and flus. Other studies of probiotics used alone or in combination with multi vitamins and minerals also found benefits in preventing colds or reducing their frequency and severity in adults.

I recommend taking lactobacilli supplements on a regular, daily basis. Adults can safely take between one billion and ten billion Lactobacilli bacteria daily, in two or more divided doses. For maximum effectiveness, take it on an empty stomach, in the morning and one hour before meals. Various cultures are available as powders, capsules, tablets, and liquids, measured by the amount of viable bacteria per dosage.

For people with dairy allergy, dairy-free formulations are available as are stabilized versions that do not require refrigeration. Be sure to check the label to confirm the recommended storage directions for the product that you have purchased. If you are currently taking antibiotics that have been prescribed by your physician for the treatment of respiratory infections, it is best to take probiotics two hours before or after taking the antibiotics.

For children under the age of 18, probiotics can also be very beneficial. For children, it is recommended to use heat-killed Lactobacillus acidophilus every twelve hours for up to five days for acute illness in dosages ranging up to a total of twelve billion organisms.

An excellent probiotic product for adults, children and even infants is Culturelle (Lactobacillus GG). In one recent study, children who received Culturelle had a significantly decreased risk of upper respiratory infections than children in the placebo group. Children with respiratory infections also recovered more quickly.

Culturelle and other probiotic products formulated for children and infants are readily available from health food stores, the Internet and Amazon.com. Other probiotic products formulated for infants and children include Child Life Essentials and Baby's Only Essentials.

Side-effects of probiotic use can include gas and bloating, although they are generally very well tolerated. If you experience these side effects, cut back on your dosage and increase slowly to your tolerance level of comfort. The use of probiotics should be avoided, however, in adults or children with significantly weakened immune systems or short bowel syndrome unless advised by your doctor.

For those people who can tolerate dairy products, soured milk products such as buttermilk, yogurt, acidophilus milk, and kefir can also be used to help restore the levels of friendly bacteria. There are also nondairy acidophilus containing products, such as soy yogurt, for people who are allergic to dairy foods.

Many small children do well on cultured food like kefir and yogurt. I have had parents tell me that their fussy children with sensitive digestive tracts are notoriously picky eaters. Often, while they may refuse to eat vegetables, meat and other important food groups, cultured foods like kefir or yogurt may be the only foods that they will eat with regularity. Additional probiotics or flaxseed oil, which is a beneficial rich source of omega 3 fatty acids, can also be added to these foods. I have seen cultured foods be very beneficial for small children.

My friend, Robin, was concerned about her infant daughter, Cynthia, who at ten months of age had frequent nasal congestion, blocked Eustachian tubes and chest congestion. She was an irritable baby who also suffered from colic, bouts of diarrhea and poor sleep. She had been treated with antibiotics that I suspected had further impacted her immunity by killing off the normal, healthy gut bacteria.

Robin had only breastfed Cynthia for a month and then had started her on commercial formula. She also fed her apple juice from a bottle. I recommended that she consider exploring the options of using donor breast milk for her infant as well as probiotics. She researched these options, talked to her regular physician and became very interested in making these changes in her infant's diet. Luckily, she was able to obtain breast milk from one of her good friends who was breastfeeding her baby as well as from other women in the community. (Donor breast milk is also available from milk banks that can be found on the Internet.) The donor breast milk and acidophilus helped greatly and her baby went from sickly to being a much healthier infant.

Colostrum

Colostrum is the first milk produced by all mammals after delivery of the newborn. While maternal milk provides important nutrients that are needed for growth and development, colostrum is crucial to the newborn's health since it enhances immunity.

Studies have shown that breast-fed human infants have better resistance to a variety of diseases, including respiratory illnesses, than bottle-fed ones. This is because colostrum contains cytokines and other low molecular weight protein compounds that act as biologic response modulators. These substances have profound anti-inflammatory and immunity-enhancing effects.

In one study published in the *British Medical Journal*, samples of human colostrum were examined and all contained respiratory virus neutralizing benefits. Immunoglobulin IgA was found in 18 out of 21 samples. IgA is known to confer protection against upper respiratory infections. This same study also found that breastfeeding conferred significant protection against respiratory illness in infants. Far fewer breast fed infants were admitted to a hospital with severe respiratory illness versus non breast fed infants.

In another research study published in *Pediatrics*, infants in Bangladesh were followed from birth to twelve months of age. Exclusive breastfeeding in these infants was found to confer significant protection against death from acute respiratory illnesses as well as death from diarrhea.

Breastfed infants also have a lower risk of middle-ear infection, which is an incredible health benefit. In a research study done at the State University of New York's School of Medicine, exclusively breastfed infants had far fewer first ear infections between the ages of six to twelve months than infants who were formula fed.

This enhanced immunity is one reason why breastfeeding is so beneficial for infants. I recommend that every mother breast feed her child until at least one year of age, if at all possible. I have seen a number of infants below the age of a year and a half with frequent respiratory infections. Often, these infants have been fed commercial formulas instead of breast milk, either from birth or because the mother discontinued breast feeding after a month or two.

A study was reported at the Rajiv Gandhi University of Health Sciences in India on the use of bovine colostrum in preventing respiratory infections in 605 children ages one through eight years old. These children were at high risk, having already suffered recurrent episodes of respiratory infections.

They were given bovine colostrum for twelve weeks and were evaluated every four weeks for episodes of recurrent infections, hospitalization, and overall well-being. At the end of the study, the episodes of recurrent respiratory infections had decreased significantly by 91% and children were overall healthier.

A study published in 2011 found that children with deficient secretory IgA had a lower severity of respiratory infections when given bovine colostrum after one week of treatment. Secretory IgA is an antibody that protects mucosal surfaces. Other studies have found that bovine colostrum can reduce symptoms and shorten the recovery time in children with diarrhea.

Adults can benefit from colostrum supplementation. In a research study published in the *European Journal of Nutrition*, bovine colostrum appeared to prevent upper respiratory infections in adult men, again probably through increasing immunoglobulins, specifically salivary IgA. It is also used in the treatment of other diseases such as rheumatoid arthritis, endometriosis, prostatitis, gluten intolerance, allergies, and herpes simplex infection.

While human colostrum is not readily available and is very expensive, concentrated derivatives of bovine colostrum are available in health food stores or from the Internet. Colostrum should be collected from the first hours of lactation. Bovine colostrum supplements are available in either a spray or a chewable enzyme.

Suggested Dosage: Use as a spray or lozenge twice a day. The product is usually held in the mouth for a minute or two to promote absorption through the mucosal lining. It is also available as capsules. Treatment times vary between two weeks and six months. For adults, the recommended dosage is 400-500 mg. taken one to three times per day as a capsule, tablet or powder. Doses as high as 10 to 20 g. have been used in research studies.

For infants and small children, it is best to get colostrum through breastfeeding or from a donor milk bank. If supplementation is necessary, several products are available. The best quality colostrum comes from New Zealand cows. Pro-Life, a New Zealand company, has developed a children's colostrum product for use in children from ages 3 years and older. They recommend chewing 1-2 tablets twice daily for children from 3 to 7 years old and 2-4 tablets per day for children 8 years and older. This product is available at shopnewzealand.co.nz

Child Life Essentials Probiotics with Colostrum is a unique combination product recommended for infants and small children. Symbiotics also produces high quality colostrum products for both adults and children. Their Symbiotics Colostrum Plus Powder and Symbiotics Colostrum Plus Chewables are both available for children. These products can be ordered through the Internet as well as Amazon.com.

Thymus Glandular Extracts

Glandular therapy involves the use of purified extracts from the secretory endocrine glands of animals. Most commonly, extracts are drawn from the thyroid and adrenal glands, as well as the thymus, pituitary, pancreas, and ovaries. Most extracts come from cows, with the exception of pancreatic glandular preparations usually drawn from sheep.

There are four common ways to extract glandulars. The first involves quick-freezing the material, washing it with a potent solvent to remove fatty tissues, distilling the solvent out, drying it, and then grinding it into a fine powder that is then encapsulated or pressed into tablets.

The second mixes freshly crushed material with salt and water that also removes fatty tissues. It is then dried and ground into a fine powder to be placed in capsules or made into tablets.

In the third method, the glandular material is freeze-dried, then placed into a vacuum chamber to remove the water. It is then encapsulated. However, with this method, fatty tissues remain.

The final method uses plant and animal enzymes to partially "digest" the material. It is then passed through a filter that separates out the fat soluble molecules. The remaining material is then freeze-dried. This method seems to be quite effective. Due to the "predigestion" all biologically active substances remain intact and can be used therapeutically to support and restore your body's endocrine glands. Healthier endocrine glands are more likely to have healthier hormone production and to be more balanced.

In the past, most experts believed that glandulars could not be effective because the intestinal lining of a healthy person was impenetrable, and that proteins and large peptides could not breach its barrier. However, recent evidence has shown that large macromolecules can and do pass completely intact from the intestinal tract into the bloodstream. In fact, there's further evidence to suggest that your body is able to determine which molecules it needs to absorb whole, and which can be broken down.

Both animal and human studies have proven this theory. In some cases, several whole proteins taken orally, including critical enzymes, have been absorbed intact into the bloodstream. Additionally, many smaller proteins and numerous hormones have also been absorbed intact into the bloodstream, including thyroid, cortisone, and even insulin.

In essence, this means that the active properties of the glandulars stay active and intact, and are not destroyed in the digestive process. This is key to the success of glandular therapy, and explains why they clearly help to restore hormone function by supporting the health of your endocrine glands themselves.

A substantial amount of clinical data now supports the effectiveness of using thymus glandular extracts. The thymus is a gland located under the breastbone and plays an important role in immune function. Thymus glandular extracts can provide benefits to people suffering from chronic viral infections and low immune function. Double-blind studies have shown that orally administrated thymus extracts can help to eliminate infection. In addition, treatment also decreased the number of respiratory infections and improved numerous immune parameters. In one small double-blind study of children with frequent respiratory infections, thymus extract reduced the rate of infections.

Thymus glandular extracts work by helping to bring T-cells (lymphocytes or white blood cells which support our immunity) into balance. They help to support T cell production when needed to help fight infections like cold, flus and lung infections, but will lower T-cell numbers in the presence of an autoimmune disease.

There are multi and single glandular systems available from companies like Standard Process—a leader in the field. However, they do require a prescription from a health care practitioner. Other good products are also available in health food stores and should be used as part of a nutritional program to support healthy menstruation.

Suggested Dosage: Take 250-500 mg once to three times a day with meals. The proper dosage of thymus extract for use in children has currently not been determined.

Echinacea

Echinacea root has long been used in traditional botanical medicine for its immunity-enhancing properties. In recent years, a number of studies have confirmed the beneficial effects that echinacea has on immune response, particularly against respiratory conditions like colds and flus.

Research studies have found that using echinacea increases phagocytosis (the process by which cells of the immune system engulf and destroy pathogenic organisms), activates macrophages to destroy pathogenic organisms, and stimulates both T lymphocytes and B lymphocytes.

In a review article published in the *European Journal of Herbal Medicine,* the author summarized the findings of six clinical trials using echinacea for the treatment of colds and flus as well as six trials that evaluated echinacea for its preventive benefits. The results of these trials confirmed that echinacea improves immune function when used for the treatment of respiratory infections.

Suggested Dosage: Take 500 to 1000 mg of echinacea in capsule form three times a day for up to five to seven days. Echinacea extract can be taken as a 300 to 800 mg. dosage two to three times a day for up to six months.

Children below the age of teenagers should take half the adult dose. Children under the age of four should take one quarter of the adult dose. Echinacea is usually safe in children from ages 2 to 11 when used for up to 10 days but note that some children might develop a rash or an allergic response.

Oregano

Oregano is a delicious culinary herb that is commonly used in Italian cuisine in the United States. It is used in such popular foods as pizza, spaghetti, and other tomato sauce based dishes. It became popular in the United States during World War II when many soldiers stationed in Europe tasted dishes made with this herb while in Italy. Oregano is also used in other cuisines, including Middle Eastern, Greek, Spanish, Portuguese and Latin American countries.

Oregano's medicinal properties were recognized as far back as the Ancient Greeks. Hippocrates used oregano as a treatment for respiratory ailments, so its usefulness in the treatment of colds, flus and lung infections goes far back in history. It has also been shown to have antimicrobial benefits against strains of Listeria monocytogenes, a food-born pathogen.

Oil of oregano is commonly used to treat acne, which results from skin infections caused by bacteria, candida infections, parasitic infections, and colds and sore throats. It is also used to treat mild indigestion which may have some basis in animal studies and has antioxidant benefits which have been confirmed in several research studies. A research study done at Georgetown University Medical Center found oregano oil to be useful in fighting yeast infections. A second study done by the same research team found it to be effective against staphylococcus aureus, a dangerous bacteria. Further research has shown it to be effective against the coronaviruses, which cause respiratory infections.

Suggested Dosage: Take 1 to 2 drops of the oil one to three times a day under the tongue. It is best to dilute oregano oil with olive oil. Side effects are rare and can include skin rashes and anaphylactic shock. It is probably safe for use in children over the age of five but shouldn't be used in infants. Consult with your health care provider about the advisability on using oil of oregano for your child, if you are interested in this therapy.

Garlic

Garlic is a delicious and pungent culinary herb, used throughout the world. It is renowned for its strong aroma and flavor. Besides being an important component of American and European cooking, garlic is also commonly used in the cuisines of the Middle East, Asia, northern Africa, and parts of South and Central America. Its use goes back to ancient Egypt during the times of the building of the pyramids and the ancient Greeks.

In modern times, entire festivals, like the Gilroy Garlic Festival in California, the Minnesota Garlic Festival and Pocono Garlic Festival in Pennsylvania are held each year. These, and many other festivals in different parts of the country, are dedicated to garlic used in every possible type of dish including garlic ice cream!

Garlic bulbs are primarily used in recipes and become more mellow and sweeter with cooking. Some recipes, like dips such as hummus or baba ghanoush, often use raw garlic to give a sweet and tangy flavor to the dishes. Olive oil, and other oils, can be infused with garlic and used in cooking.

Garlic cloves are also used raw, dried or cooked for their medicinal benefits. Garlic contains an organic compound, called allicin, which gives garlic its aroma and flavor and is also a very powerful antioxidant.

Research published in the chemistry journal *Angewandte Chemie* found that allicin is a very powerful and rapid acting antioxidant that destroys dangerous free radicals. This reaction occurs once allicin decomposes and produces an acid that powerfully reacts with free radicals. Although onions, leeks and shallots are in the same plant family as garlic and contain a compound similar to allicin, they do not have the same medicinal properties.

Garlic has a long history of use as an antimicrobial agent. In World War I and World War II, garlic was used as an antiseptic and antimicrobial agent to help prevent gangrene A mouthwash containing fresh garlic was developed that showed antimicrobial activity. However, most of the study participants did not like the mouthwash because it had an unpleasant taste and caused bad smelling breath.

In in vitro studies, garlic has been found to have antimicrobial properties. Studies have shown garlic to have antibacterial, antiviral and antifungal activity. It is often used to treat candida infections and thrush, a fungal infection of the throat. People also use garlic to prevent and treat the common cold and sinus infections.

A review of data done by the University of Alberta, Canada and published in *Pediatrics in Review* found that children had better results from taking garlic tablets for respiratory infections than from taking medication or placebo.

When applied topically in combination with mullein in oil-based products, it has been found to reduce the pain, but not the actual infection, of otitis media or middle ear infections. However, the topical use of garlic may cause burning or blistering of the skin in some sensitive individuals so it should be used carefully.

Suggested Dosage: When using raw garlic, 4 grams of fresh garlic per day (approximately 1 clove) may be effective. Garlic capsules are also avail-able, including deodorized garlic, which is more readily tolerated by many people. Suggested dosage of garlic is 900 mg per day of a garlic powder standardized to contain 1.3% allicin. Garlic may also be found in cream or oil products for topical use.

The recommendations for use of deodorized garlic in children from Kyolic, a prominent manufacturer is:

Ages 1-6 months: Start out with 1-2 drops in liquid (formula, juice or water) once a day for 1-2 weeks. If well tolerated, dosage may be gradually increased to about ¼ tsp. a day.

Ages 6-18 months: Start out with 2-3 drops in liquid once a day for 1-2 weeks. If well tolerated, the dosage may be gradually increased to about ¼ to ½ tsp. a day.

Ages 18 months-3 years: Start out with 3-4 drops in liquid once a day for 1-2 weeks. If well tolerated, the dosage may be gradually increased to about ¼ to ½ tsp. a day.

Ages older than 3 years: Start out with ¼ tsp once a day for 1-2 weeks. If well tolerated, the dosage may be gradually increased to about ½ to ¾ tsp a day.

After an infant has been taking Kyolic for a time, the liquid may be put into his food, instead of his liquids. Also, the total daily amount may be given all at one time or divided into two or more servings.

The most common side effect of garlic use is body odor, bad breath and a burning sensation in the mouth. Some people report having heartburn or diarrhea with the use of raw garlic and find that they cannot tolerate it. Garlic use should also be avoided by people on anticoagulant drugs like Coumadin because of its blood thinning properties.

It is possibly safe for pregnant and nursing mothers except just before and immediately after delivery, although this has not been definitely proven. If you have any questions or concerns, I recommend that you ask your doctor about the advisability of using garlic for your particular case.

Ginseng

Ginseng root has been used as a tonic to improve resistance to disease in traditional Asian medicine for several thousand years. Research studies have confirmed that ginseng root improves immune function by stimulating the activity of natural killer cells and increasing the production of lymphocytes.

An article published in *Drugs Under Experimental and Clinical Research* discussed the results of a study in which the ability of ginseng to improve immune response to the influenza vaccine was evaluated versus a placebo.

Two hundred twenty-seven adult volunteers were given either 100 mg of a standardized extract of ginseng root or a placebo daily over a twelve-week period. All of the volunteers were given an influenza vaccine at week four.

The volunteers taking the ginseng root showed a significantly greater immune response to the influenza vaccine than did the placebo group. In addition, the individuals in the treatment group experienced fewer cases of influenza and fewer colds than those in the placebo group.

Suggested Dosage: For maximum benefit, take a high-quality preparation, an extract of the main root of a plant that is four to six years old, standardized for ginsenoside content and ratio. Twice a day, take a 100 mg capsule. If this is too stimulating, especially before bedtime, take the second dose midafternoon, or take only the morning dose. I do not recommend the use of ginseng in infants and children for treating respiratory infections.

Vitamins and Minerals

For both adults and children who are prone to colds, flus, and respiratory infections, I recommend supplementing with multi-nutrient product. For children, you should use a high quality product specifically formulated for this age group that is abundant in the nutrients vitamins C, B complex, D, and zinc and follow the directions on the label. This will help to boost immunity and resistance to infections and support all around health and well being in people of all ages.

Good products for kids include Nature's Plus - Animal Parade Baby Plex Multi, Yummi Bears Multi-Vitamin and Mineral, and Country Life Dolphin Pals DHA Gummies for Kids, for anti-inflammatory omega 3 fatty acids. There are many other similar, high quality brands for children. I am not partial, however, to many of the mass market products found on your grocery store and pharmacy shelves that tend to be of a lesser quality.

The benefits of multi-nutrients for children were reinforced in a study published in the *International Journal of Pediatric Otorhinolaryngology* (quite a mouthful to say, but this essentially refers to medical research of the ears, nose and throat in children). This study looked at young children with chronic, recurrent sinusitis. The children, who ranged from 4.2 to 9.8 years of age, were given lemon-flavored cod liver oil and a children's multivitamin/multimineral product. The study went on for several months and the children on these supplements were found to have a reduction in their symptoms of sinusitis, fewer episodes of sinusitis and fewer doctor visits. This is very exciting news for parents!

In addition, there are certain specific nutrients that are very useful for the treatment of cold, flus, and other respiratory infections that need to be used at higher dosages than are often found in a multi. You may want to use them at the recommended dosages in addition to the multi-nutrient. These nutrients include:

Vitamin C and Bioflavonoids

Vitamin C and bioflavonoids have anti-inflammatory properties and help to reduce the course of a cold. Although they do not "cure" the common cold, the infectious process can be less severe.

Suggested Dosage: I recommend 500 to 1,000 milligrams of mineral buffered (alkaline) vitamin C and bioflavonoids three to four times a day. If you develop loose stools, reduce the amount and frequency of these supplements.

If your child is prone to colds or other respiratory infections, you may want to boost their intake of vitamin C since it may reduce the duration of the illness. Vitamin C products formulated for children include Child Life Essentials Liquid Vitamin C and Natures Plus Animal Parade Vitamin C Orange Juice Flavor. The vitamin C products tend to be between 100 to 250 mg per serving.

The Child Life product is 250 mg per serving and recommends one-quarter teaspoon for infants 6 months to 1 year and one half to one teaspoon for children one to four years old.

Pantothenic Acid

Pantothenic acid supports adrenal function, which is often compromised when you have a cold. It also helps to minimize nasal congestion and fatigue.

Suggested Dosage: I recommend 250 milligrams two to three times daily for up to one week for adults. It should be taken with a vitamin B complex so that you receive the support of the entire family of B vitamins.

Vitamin D

Current research suggests that one reason for the widespread frequency of colds, flus, and respiratory infections in the U.S. is that vitamin D deficiency is common during the winter when these infections are at their peak. A number of studies have shown that there is an inverse relationship between respiratory infections and vitamin D levels within the body. One study found that people with the lowest levels of vitamin D have many more cases of colds and flus. Research on vitamin D levels and flu in children found similar results.

Suggested Dosage: I recommend 10,000 IU of vitamin D supplement per day for adults, especially during the winter cold and flu season. Children need approximately 35 IU's of vitamin D per pound of body weight.

Zinc

Zinc appears to be most beneficial for the treatment of colds when taken within 24 hours of the onset of the infection. Zinc taken during this time appears to reduce the duration and severity of cold symptoms. While research studies are inconclusive, patients do find that it also helps to sooth a sore throat.

Suggested Dosage: Take 5 to 10 milligrams of zinc in lozenge form every three hours, to a total of 50 milligrams daily, for three days. Alternatively, take 50 to 75 milligrams of supplemental zinc per day while fighting a cold. For children under the age of eighteen, similar dosages have been recommended taken as a lozenge.

Remember Sarah, the five-year-old girl, whose story I shared with you in the first chapter? This is her current nutritional supplement program that is keeping her cold and earache free. I am sharing this with you as a sample program that I have seen work very well with children:

- Dolphin Pals DHA by Country Life
- Yummi Bears Multi-Vitamin & Minerals by Hero
- Buddy Bear Probiotics by Renew Life
- Buddy Bear Digestive Enzymes by Renew Life
- Silver Biotics colloidal silver product if she begins to show any signs of a cold to "nip it in the bud" so that the cold never develops.

6

The Importance of Acid/Alkaline Balance

Acid/alkaline balance or having a healthy pH plays a major role not only in preventing colds, flus and lung infections but in assisting with rapid recovery. This is an essential part of your program and will create great benefits not only in eliminating respiratory infections but for your health in general, if followed carefully. Let me explain what pH means a little further.

Understanding pH

All substances in nature can be classified according to their relative acidity or alkalinity. The origin of the word acid is the Latin word "acidus", which means sour or tart. These qualities characterize many of the common acidic substances that we come in contact with, such as the vinegar used in salad dressings, which contain acetic acid; soft drinks, which contain phosphoric acid and carbon dioxide; and black tea, which contains tannic acid. Citric acid is found in grapefruits, oranges, lemons, and limes; and tartaric acid comes from grapes.

In contrast, alkaline substances have a bitter taste and feel slippery or smooth on the tongue. A good example is sodium bicarbonate, also known as baking soda, which is used as an antacid.

The acidity and alkalinity of all substances are expressed in terms of pH, which measures the concentration of hydrogen ions. A pH ranking above 7.00 indicates that a substance is alkaline, and below 7.00 is acidic. Pure water has a pH close to neutral, or 7.00.

The pH measurement is an extremely sensitive calibration, with an increase or decrease from one whole number to another indicating a tenfold increase or decrease in hydrogen ion concentration. Thus, seemingly small shifts in the pH value of a substance can reflect significant changes in its relative acidity or alkalinity.

How pH Functions Within Your Body

Your body contains trillions of cells, fluid-filled structures that contain many alkaline substances: minerals such as calcium, magnesium, potassium, and sodium, as well as oxygen and bicarbonate. The combination of all of these substances within the cell produces a slightly alkaline intracellular pH of just above 7.00. The cells are also surrounded by fluids that contain alkaline minerals.

Not only are the cells of the body alkaline, but the blood that circulates throughout your body must maintain a very narrow range of slightly alkaline pH, 7.35 to 7.45. The constancy of the blood pH is fundamental to the body's ability to maintain a relatively unchanging internal environment.

The blood is constantly exposed to a variety of mostly acidic substances. Various things, from the foods you eat and the stresses in your life to the pollutants you are exposed to—as well as your own metabolic processes—produce chemicals within the body that are often more acidic than your own slightly alkaline pH.

All of these substances are carried within the blood, which transports them to the cells for use as nutrients or carries them away from the cells as waste products. All of these substances potentially disrupt the healthy pH of the blood.

As a result, your body has to have a mechanism to both neutralize and eliminate these substances in order to keep the pH of the blood constant. This is the pH-regulating system. Its importance is illustrated by the fact that a person cannot live more than a few hours if the blood's pH goes below 7.00 or above 8.00. For example, blood with a pH of 6.95, which is only slightly acidic, can lead to coma and even death.

How the Body Regulates Acid/Alkaline Balance

The pH-regulating system of the body is very complex and is made up of many parts. Within the body, the various parts of our pH-regulating system are carefully orchestrated to work well together. The system includes the alkaline minerals contained both inside and outside the cells, as well as the mineral reserves stored within our bones. We also have three buffer systems in the blood that help to keep its pH constant.

In addition, the lungs help to regulate pH by breathing in alkaline oxygen and eliminating acidic waste products in the form of carbon dioxide. Finally, the kidneys eliminate excessive amounts of either acid or alkaline substances from the body through the urine.

The pH-regulating system tends to be healthy and to work efficiently in children and young adults. There are children who have weak buffer systems and tend to become overly acidic early in life as well as some youngsters who are high-alkaline producers and maintain this tendency throughout life. The healthy buffering capability of most young people is due to the robust mineral reserves stored in their bones, healthy buffer systems, and strong lung and kidney function. However, as people age and experience the mostly acidifying stresses of modern life, the pH-regulating system begins to decline in its efficiency.

This decline is a part of the normal aging process and can be accelerated by such factors as strenuous athletic activity or years of acidifying stress or of eating the standard Western diet. As a result, with age, more and more individuals who formerly had good pH balance tend to become overly acidic. Over acidity increases our susceptibility to many diseases including infections, inflammatory diseases and even cancer.

Over Acidity Makes Us More Susceptible to Colds, Flus and Lung Infections

The most common health-related success saboteurs in our society today are minor respiratory illnesses. When the body is overly acidic, a person is often much more susceptible to such ailments as colds, flus, bronchitis, sinusitis, middle ear infections and even pneumonia. The bacteria and viruses that cause these infections thrive in low-oxygen, acidic environments. For most people with these conditions, restoring your body rapidly to a more healthful, slightly alkaline state is one of the most important steps that you can take to recover rapidly.

Over acidity, due to a highly acidic diet, emotional stress, or poor oxygenation, makes a person more susceptible to respiratory infections. The symptoms of respiratory illnesses, sneezing, sore throats, runny noses, sinusitis, middle ear infections, and coughing, worsen as an individual becomes increasingly more acidic.

In the more serious cases of respiratory infection, such as severe pneumonia, affected individuals can even develop respiratory acidosis, a potentially life-threatening condition in which the pH of the blood drops to dangerously low levels, and the lungs are no longer able to ventilate properly and make the necessary pH corrections by eliminating carbon dioxide from the body.

To rapidly suppress a respiratory infection, I recommend beginning an alkalinization program at the first sign of symptoms. Alkalinizing agents can be tremendously beneficial in assisting the body to rapidly neutralize over acidity and bring very fast relief from symptoms of colds, flus, and lung infections. These agents can rapidly catalyze a shift from over acidity to a healthier, more alkaline state. The almost immediate relief that alkalinizing substances can provide makes them an extremely powerful part of any program to rapidly recover from colds, flus, and lung infections.

Sodium Bicarbonate

Sodium bicarbonate is the most powerful and rapid acting alkalinizing substance for the treatment of colds, flus and lung infections. It is a nontoxic, white crystalline powder that has a mild, neutral taste. It is also referred to as baking soda and bicarbonate of soda.

Baking soda is identical to the buffering substance produced within our own body and is one of the most powerful, and effective alkalinizing agents. It works very rapidly to help reduce symptoms of colds, flus and lung infections. I have seen numerous patients who suffer from respiratory infections benefit greatly from its use. As a buffering agent, sodium bicarbonate easily reacts with other compounds and produces a significantly alkaline end product with a pH of 8.1.

Not only is sodium bicarbonate an essential part of the buffer system of our body, it is also active in the natural ecology of the Earth. Sodium bicarbonate plays a role in maintaining the pH balance in all living things. It is found in lake sediments, mineral deposits, groundwater, and even the ocean, where it helps stabilize the amount of carbon dioxide in the atmosphere.

Suggested Dosage: To treat a respiratory ailment in the acute stage (from the first sign or symptom), take one-half to one teaspoon of sodium bicarbonate on an empty stomach. Sodium bicarbonate should not be taken right after eating as it may interfere with the early phase digestion of protein and other foods.

You may need to use sodium bicarbonate every few hours for a short period of time until your symptoms start to diminish. At this point, dosages can be spread out to every three to four hours while the person is still in the acute phase of the illness. In contrast, an individual with mild sinusitis may find that using bicarbonate once or twice a day on a daily basis provides enough buffering to prevent their symptoms from occurring. Do NOT, however, take more than 5-6 doses total in a day.

I recommend taking one dose before going to bed and another upon rising in the morning. During the acute phase, you may even take the bicarbonate mixture every few hours during the night. Acids tend to accumulate during the night, and a person with relatively few symptoms the night before may wake the next day with a return of their congestion.

In the acute stages of a respiratory infection, it's a good idea to prepare a solution of sodium bicarbonate and water in a closed container and keep it next to the bed so that you can sip on it whenever you wake up or go to the bathroom. This will allow for more continuous alkalinizing of the body that is necessary to restore the environment needed for the body to control and eliminate the bacteria or viruses that are causing the symptoms. Also, be sure to continue the alkalinizing process for several days after the acute symptoms have subsided to prevent a recurrence of your symptoms.

If you are concerned about taking large dosages of sodium bicarbonate because of a need to limit your sodium intake because of high blood pressure or a history of congestive heart failure, you may want to use a combination of sodium and potassium bicarbonate, instead. It is also not recommended for women who are pregnant.

Children have special recommendations for sodium bicarbonate. Firstly, sodium bicarbonate should not be given to children under the age of six unless approved by your health care provider. Children from 6 to 12 years old can be given one quarter to one half teaspoon of sodium bicarbonate mixed in water per dosage. Children in this age group and older can often benefit from sodium bicarbonate if they have recurrent colds, flus, middle ear infections, and sinus and chest congestion since they may be overly acidic. The dietary recommendations for the alkaline power diet further on in this chapter can also be very helpful for both adults and children.

Potassium Bicarbonate

Potassium bicarbonate can be purchased readily on the Internet and in some health food stores as a nutritional supplement product. A pharmacist can also prepare a mixture of sodium bicarbonate and potassium bicarbonate, or an individual can make his or her own sodium and potassium bicarbonate mixture. Like sodium bicarbonate, potassium bicarbonate is a white, crystalline, nontoxic powder. Both substances will last indefinitely if stored in a cool, dry place.

However, while sodium bicarbonate has a mild, pleasant taste, potassium bicarbonate is somewhat sharp and chalky on the tongue. Potassium bicarbonate is rarely taken alone because of its unpalatable taste.

Sodium and Potassium Bicarbonate Combinations

Some people prefer to use sodium and potassium in combination in a ratio of 3:1 to 4:1 sodium to potassium (depending on your tolerance for potassium) rather than using sodium bicarbonate alone to treat colds, flus and lung infections.

There are some benefits to using both sodium and potassium bicarbonate in a mixture. First of all, the digestive juices produced by the pancreas contain both sodium and potassium. In addition, many individuals do not eat enough potassium-rich foods in their diet. There are also other health benefits to supplementing with both buffering agents since this helps to maintain the sodium-potassium balance of the cells.

For a cell to be healthy, there must be a predominance of potassium inside the cell and sodium outside it. This condition generates an electrical charge that allows the cell wall to control which substances enter the cell and to discharge toxins from the cell. Since the standard American diet contains an overabundance of sodium and is low in potassium (commonly supplied by fresh plant foods), our diet itself can potentially disturb the important balance of these intracellular and extracellular minerals.

However, there are individuals who do find potassium bicarbonate irritating to their digestive tract or have a preexisting health condition for which the use of a potassium-based supplement is contraindicated. Furthermore, if taken alone in a high dosage for prolonged periods of time, it may cause an irregular heartbeat. Such individuals can use sodium bicarbonate alone as an alkalinizing agent. See your physician if you have any specific questions.

When treating respiratory infections, it is important that you do not stop alkalinizing prematurely since these overly acidic condition may not have been completely neutralized and symptoms may recur.

Occasionally, an individual will find that he or she needs to go as high as a one-teaspoon dosage for short periods of time in order to relieve their symptoms. Conversely, very sensitive individuals may find that a tiny dose, such as one-eighth teaspoon, is sufficient.

How Long Should I Continue to Use Alkalinizing Agents?

Physicians who work with nutritional programs to restore acid/alkaline balance often find that highly acidic people may need to use sodium and potassium bicarbonate on a more regular basis, even for as long as several years. Higher dosages may be necessary during the first four to six months of treatment to counteract their chronic over acidity. The dosages can gradually be reduced, except during periods of great physical or emotional stress, when higher dosages may be necessary.

At the same time, however, these physicians will often place their patients on more alkalinizing diets and alkaline mineral supplementation, both of which are needed to build up the alkaline reserves of the body and counteract over acidity. Alkaline minerals include calcium, magnesium, potassium and zinc. A high potency multivitamin and multimineral product should provide adequate levels of these essential nutrients.

The use of alkalinizing agents alone on a long-term basis will not produce maximum therapeutic benefits unless these other restorative steps are followed so that the healthful, slightly alkaline pH of the body can be restored.

However, in order to restore major body systems that are greatly overly acidic and to offset the over acidity that develops as part of the normal aging process, an individual (particularly if past midlife) may have to continue a maintenance program of alkalinizing agents for a prolonged period of time or even indefinitely.

It is always helpful to begin any program to restore your acid/alkaline balance with the help of either a physician who is knowledgeable about nutritional medicine or a well-trained nutritionist.

A Caution on Taking Bicarbonate of Soda

Very occasionally, a person will use too much bicarbonate and become overly alkaline. If this occurs, you may experience any of several symptoms, including a tingling sensation in the extremities, feeling over energized, being unable to sleep, and, rarely, muscle spasms. If you should experience any of these symptoms, immediately discontinue use of the bicarbonate. Acidifying the system with a teaspoon or two of cider vinegar or the juice of half a lemon in water will help to neutralize the excess alkalinity.

You can try instituting treatment again the following day, but at a lower dosage and at less frequent intervals. If symptoms are severe, you may want to consult with your physician as to the advisability of using bicarbonate therapy at all for your particular case.

The Most Appropriate Dosages for Your Age: from Childhood to Old Age

While the dosages provided in this chapter are appropriate for most people, there are certain groups who should use less than the recommended dosages, as previously mentioned.

Children, the elderly, and individuals with a frail constitution or who are extremely sensitive to drugs and nutritional supplements usually do best at therapeutic dosages of no more than half, or even one quarter, of the recommended levels.

Consult your physician or nutritional consultant if you have any questions about the advisability of using a particular nutritional supplement or to determine the dosage most appropriate for you.

The One Exception to This Rule: High-alkaline Producers and Respiratory Illnesses

In contrast to the rest of us, some individuals who are naturally high-alkaline producers tend to be more resistant to respiratory illnesses.

How do you identify if you are a high alkaline producer? These are individuals that tend to have strong alkaline reserves within their bodies such as their bones and other tissues and have strong buffering capacity. They tend to have larger, denser bones and muscles, healthy digestive function, strong immunity, and excellent resistance to disease.

If they do come down with a cold or flu, over acidity is usually not the trigger. Often, other factors such as liver toxicity or diminished production of anti-inflammatory digestive enzymes or stress hormones may increase their susceptibility to respiratory infection.

If these naturally alkaline individuals do come down with a cold or flu, they tend to recover quickly. They will leave work for a half day or a day, take a nap, eat lightly, and bounce right back. Interestingly, people with very effectively functioning systems have no idea why they are this way.

A good example of these disease resistant types is physicians. Most family-practice doctors and pediatricians are exposed to respiratory infections from their patients on a regular basis. However, physicians tend to have hearty, alkaline constitutions; a prerequisite if a young doctor is to survive the rigors of the medical training process.

If you are a high-alkaline producer and develop a respiratory condition, then the old-fashioned remedy of orange juice and Jell-O *is* just what you need. Do not use alkalinizing agents since they will tend to over-alkalinize you and will probably worsen your symptoms. Your condition is probably due to a chemical imbalance other than pH. In your case, the anti-inflammatory therapies, oxygen therapies, and detoxification therapies described in my other books would probably be most helpful in treating a respiratory infection.

Two Alkaline pH Success Stories

I want to share two stories of how my pH balancing program saved the day for both myself and my patient, Robert. Each of us has a story of how rapid treatment of respiratory infections with alkalinizing agents saved the day. The use of alkalinizing agents allowed us to resume our normal schedules very rapidly, despite the onset of severe respiratory symptoms. These infections would normally have caused us to be ill and functioning inefficiently for as long as two to three weeks.

Roberta's Story. Since learning how to restore my acid/alkaline balance in my forties through working with Dr. Lark's program, I have been able to prevent the onset of or easily contain the symptoms of colds, flus, sinusitis, and bronchitis. These problems had plagued me since my early-childhood days. I am now able to eliminate these infections the way all naturally alkaline peak performers do.

However, since I am not one of those individuals, I must always be ready to counter any tendency toward over acidity that can occur if I overstress my body beyond its normal pH tolerances. If you are like me and tend toward over acidity, the following story will show you the importance of always having a fully stocked alkalinizing kit available when traveling.

Several years ago, I scheduled a multicity cross-country trip, in mid-summer, to close a business deal that I had been working on for many months. Halfway into the scheduled ten-day trip, I realized it would have to be extended for at least another week. This meant more hotel living, airplane flights, and entertaining the potential business partners with rich foods and, often, too many cocktails and wine with dinner.

The last city on the itinerary was New Orleans. Due to a shortage of rooms, I was given a room reserved for smokers (I have never smoked) that had been treated with toxic chemicals in an attempt to remove the smell of cigarette smoke. On top of that, the air conditioner's thermostat was set very low to combat the New Orleans summer heat and could not be adjusted by the hotel engineer.

The unhealthy conditions at the hotel plus the stress of travel, too much work, and all the rich food and drink sent me into a violently over-acidic state. As I got on the plane to return to San Francisco, I knew I was coming down with something. Due to the length of the trip, I had used up my alkalinizing travel kit and sat on the six-hour flight without any emergency supplies.

During the flight, I developed a sore throat, and my nose began to run. When I arrived home, I felt weak and was sneezing, coughing, and shaking with the chills, even though it was July. I immediately began an accelerated alkalinizing program, rested, and dramatically reduced my food intake. Within a few days, I was well on the road to recovery.

My Story. Several years ago, I pushed myself beyond my limits when I accepted numerous teaching engagements all over the state of California and was also completing several professional projects. I worked almost two months without a break, with relatively little sleep each night.

Toward the end of the second month, I was driving to a weekend seminar where I was the featured lecturer. On the way, to the seminar, I stopped at a deli where I ate a very acidic meal consisting of salads and vegetables that seemed to be marinated in pure vinegar.

The acidity of the meal coupled with my high level of work-related stress finally threw me into a state of extreme over acidity. As soon as I left the deli, I began to have a runny nose and couldn't stop sneezing. This occurred six hours before I was due to give my first lecture.

Fortunately, I had brought my buffering agents and supplements with me, as I usually do in case of an emergency. I started taking sodium and potassium bicarbonate every half hour for the first several hours, and then continued this regimen every hour. I also began to take digestive enzymes and buffered vitamin C to reduce the inflammation.

After five hours of alkalinizing myself, I had restored my pH balance. My sneezing stopped, and the congestion cleared up almost entirely. I was able to meet my responsibilities and teach for the entire weekend, but I continued to use these alkalinizing agents to avoid a relapse. Given how tired and stressed I was, there is no question that without these lifesavers I would have begun a downward spiral and spent a number of days in bed. By restoring my pH balance, however, I was able to get through a very busy weekend and continue with my normal schedule on Monday.

Business travel and lavish vacations create the perfect conditions for becoming overly acidic. Unless you are a high-alkaline producer, it's a good idea to take an emergency alkalinizing kit to ward off colds and flus when traveling for business or pleasure. The kit should contain an alkalinizing agent, buffered vitamin C, alkaline minerals, herbs such as ginger or curcumin with aspirin-like properties, and anti-inflammatory digestive enzymes. These are discussed in the following chapters of this book.

Follow the Alkaline Power Diet

If you tend toward frequent respiratory infections, it is important that you follow on an on-going basis a more alkaline diet and greatly reduce the intake of highly acidic foods in your diet. My alkaline power diet will help to restore you to a naturally healthy state of slight alkalinity that will support your immunity and improve your resistance to respiratory infections. By avoiding highly acidic foods and eating foods that are neutral to slightly alkaline in their pH, you will restore your reserves of alkaline minerals and other important nutrients.

Equally important, this diet will decrease the wear and tear on your buffer systems and organs of elimination by reducing the acid load of the body. This diet will cause fewer inflammatory reactions, which are extremely acidifying to the cells and tissues and predispose you towards colds, flus, sinusitis, middle ear infections and lung infections.

Selecting the Proper Foods for the Alkaline Power Diet

First, look at the following chart showing the pH values of dozens of common foods and beverages. This chart will help you to learn the relative acidity or alkalinity of the foods that most of us eat on a daily basis. (You may be surprised at how acidic many of the foods you currently eat are.)

It gives the pH of foods prior to being consumed and does not reflect the substantial acid production that some of these foods can trigger within the body. (Information on this topic is also provided in this section.)

There is a lot of misinformation about the relative acidity and alkalinity of foods. Many other books have acid/alkaline food charts; however, these charts tend to contradict one another. One chart will list a food as being highly acidic, while another chart will state that the same food is highly alkaline. This can be very confusing to the reader who is trying to use this information to make intelligent choices.

My chart is based on scientific research done at major universities. This information was obtained from technical sources compiled at the University of California, Davis, Department of Food Science and Technology, and Cornell University, Department of Food Science. In addition, I obtained the pH value of

pH of Common Foods and Beverage
Prior to Being Consumed

Highly Acidic Foods	pH Range (pH between 1 and 4.6)
Beverages	
Ginger ale	2.0–4.0
Lime juice	2.2–2.4
Lemon juice	2.2–2.6
Wines	2.3–3.8
Cranberry juice	2.5–2.7
Cider	2.9–3.3

certain foods from their appropriate professional associations such as the National Coffee Association.

You will notice that while most food groups are listed, oils are not. Oils do not have a pH since they cannot be mixed with water, which is necessary for taking pH measurements. Many books will list the pH for oils. Which is totally incorrect!

The chart will help you to plan a diet best suited to your pH needs, depending on whether you tend toward over acidity or are a naturally alkaline person. Overly acidic individuals can restore their bodies to a healthier, more alkaline state by using this chart to select foods that are less acidic and more alkaline. The chart will also indicate which foods have the highest level of acidity and should be avoided.

Grapefruit juice	2.9–3.4
Currant juice	3.0
Orange juice	3.0–4.0
Apple juice	3.3–3.5
Pineapple juice	3.4–3.7
Prune juice	3.7–4.3
Tomato juice	3.9–4.3
Fruit	
Lime	1.8–2.0
Lemon	2.2–2.4
Cranberry sauce	2.3
Gooseberries	2.8–3.1
Loquats	2.8–4.0
Orange	2.8–4.2
Plum	2.8–4.6
Rhubarb	2.9–3.4
Apple	2.9–3.5
Raspberries	2.9–3.7
Grapefruit	2.9–4.0
Boysenberries	3.0–3.3
Grapefruit sections	3.0–3.5
Strawberries	3.0–4.2
Blackberries	3.0–4.2
Kumquat	3.1–3.5
Quince	3.2
Blueberries	3.2–3.6
Pineapple, crushed	3.2–4.0
Crab apples, spiced	3.3–3.7
Kiwi	3.3–3.8
Apple sauce	3.4–3.5
Apricots	3.5–4.0
Pineapple, sliced	3.5–4.1
Fruit cocktail	3.6–4.0

Raisins	3.6–4.2
Vegetables	
Sauerkraut	3.1–3.7
Cucumber	3.1–3.8
Tomatillo	3.9–4.1
Dairy Products	
Yogurt	3.8–4.2
Sweeteners	
Fruit jellies	3.0–3.5
Fruit jams	3.5–4.0
Condiments and Seasonings	
Vinegar	2.4–3.4
Pickles, sweet	2.5–3.0
Pickles, dill	2.6–3.8
Pickles, sour	3.0–3.5
Fermented olives	3.5
Mayonnaise	3.8–4.0

Moderately Acidic Foods	pH Range (pH between 3.1 and 5.6)
Beverages	
Beer	4.0–5.0
Fruit	
Peach	3.1–4.7
Cherries	3.2–4.7
Pear	3.4–4.7
Mango	3.9–4.6
Asian pear	4.2–4.6
Guava	4.3–4.7
Banana	4.5–5.2

Vegetables

Tomato	3.7–4.9
Potato salad	3.9–4.6
Eggplant	4.5–4.7
String beans	4.6

Red Meat

Dry sausage	4.4–5.6

Dairy Products

Cottage cheese	4.1–5.4

Condiments and Seasonings

Fermented vegetables	3.9–5.1
Red pimento	4.3–5.2

Low Acid to Alkaline Foods	pH Range (pH between 4.6 and 9.5)
Beverages	
Coffee	4.9–5.2
Mineral water	6.2–9.4
Distilled water	6.8–7.0
Fruit	
Figs	4.6–5.0
Papaya	5.2–5.7
Persimmon	5.4–5.8
Avocado	5.5–6.0
Dates	6.2–6.4
Cantaloupe	6.2–6.5
Melon	6.3–6.7
Vegetables	
Pumpkin	4.8–5.5
Sweet pepper	4.8–6.0
Spinach	4.8–6.8

Carrot	4.9–6.3
Squash	5.0–5.4
Asparagus	5.0–6.1
Turnip	5.2–5.6
Cabbage	5.2–6.3
Broccoli	5.2–6.5
Parsnip	5.3
Sweet potato	5.3–5.6
Onion	5.3–5.8
Peas	5.3–6.8
Turnip greens	5.4–5.6
White potato	5.4–6.3
Artichoke	5.6
Cauliflower	5.6–6.7
Parsley	5.7–6.0
Celery	5.7–6.1
Alfalfa tops	5.9
Corn	5.9–7.3
Lettuce	6.0–6.4
Mushrooms	6.0–6.5
Brussels sprout	6.3–6.6
Beans	
Baked beans	4.8–5.5
Dried beans	4.9–5.5
Kidney	5.2–5.4
Lima	5.4–6.5
Soybeans	6.0–6.6
Nuts and Seeds	
Walnuts	5.4–5.5
Almonds	> 6.0
Flaxseeds	> 6.0
Hazelnuts	> 6.0
Pecans	> 6.0

Poppy seeds	> 6.0
Pumpkin seeds	> 6.0
Sesame seeds	> 6.0
Sunflower seeds	> 6.0

Fish and Shellfish

Halibut	5.5–5.8
Sardines	5.7–6.6
Tuna	5.9–6.1
Mackerel	5.9–6.2
Oysters	5.9–6.7
Clams	5.9–7.1
Codfish (canned)	6.0–6.1
Salmon	6.1–6.5
Haddock	6.2–6.7
Whiting	6.2–7.1
Catfish	6.6–7.0
Scallops	6.8–7.1
Crab	6.8–8.0
Shrimp	6.8–8.2

Poultry

Chicken	5.5–6.4
Duck	6.0–6.1
Egg yolk	6.0–6.3
Egg white	7.9–9.5

Red Meat

Beef	5.3–6.2
Pork	5.3–6.4
Corned-beef hash	5.5–6.0
Spiced ham	6.0–6.3
Hot dogs	6.2

Dairy Products

Roquefort cheese	4.7–4.8
Most cheeses	5.0–6.1
Parmesan cheese	5.2–5.3
Evaporated milk	5.9–6.3
Whole cow's milk	6.0–6.8
Butter	6.1–6.4
Camembert	6.1–7.0
Grains	
Wheat	> 6.0
Rice	> 6.0
Barley	> 6.0
Oats	> 6.0
Rye	> 6.0
Millet	> 6.0
Quinoa	> 6.0
Amaranth	> 6.0
Hominy	6.9–7.9
Baked Goods	
White bread	5.0–6.0
Date-nut bread	5.1–6.0
Soda crackers	6.5–8.5
Sweeteners	
Molasses	5.0–5.4
Glucose syrup	5.2
Honey	6.0–6.8
Brown-rice syrup	6.1–6.4
Maple syrup	6.5–7.0
Condiments and Seasonings	
Hot peppers	4.8–6.0
Garlic	5.3–6.3
Cocoa	5.5–6.0
Ripe, canned olives	5.9–7.3
Dutch processed chocolate	7.0–8.0

More About the Alkaline Diet

If you have symptoms of over acidity and are prone towards respiratory infections, it is important to eat foods listed in the "Low Acid to Alkaline" section of the chart. Eating foods such as vegetables, starches, non gluten-containing grains, legumes (beans and peas), small amounts of raw seeds and nuts, poultry, fish, shellfish, sea vegetables, and more alkaline fruits like papaya and melons will help to lessen the acid load of the body.

Low acidic foods will also reduce the wear and tear on the pH-regulating systems as well as the organs of elimination. Ground, raw flax meal deserves a special mention as a rich source of both alkaline minerals and anti-inflammatory omega 3 oils. Flax meal can be used in blender drinks and as a cereal.

If you are overly acidic, eating these foods will not only support your immunity and improve your resistance to respiratory infections like colds, flus, and lung infections but will begin to enhance your performance in many areas of your life as well as increase your physical energy, stamina, and resistance to disease. Health benefits include reducing the risk of heart attacks and strokes, cancer, and crippling, inflammatory conditions like arthritis.

The more alkaline foods are higher in essential nutrients and are full of the alkaline minerals needed to restore the alkaline reserves in your cells, tissues, and bones. These foods also tend to be less allergenic and less likely to cause inflammatory reactions, which acidify your cells.

Your diet and food selection should concentrate on foods that have a pH above 5.0. This will create a diet that has a vegetarian emphasis but includes rich sources of proteins like legumes, whole grains, raw seeds and nuts, and fish and shellfish. Fish and shellfish do not have the tough, fibrous protein found in red meat. As a result, the stomach produces less hydrochloric acid to digest these foods than is necessary for the breakdown of red meat.

Fish such as salmon, mackerel, trout, and tuna also contain anti-inflammatory polyunsaturated oils rather than the inflammatory saturated fats found in red meat and dairy products. Because of the accumulation of mercury, they should not be eaten more than twice a week. In addition, mercury free fish or algae based omega 3 oils can be taken as a supplement for daily use.

Avoid highly acidic foods and acid-forming foods

More than 90 percent of Americans become overly acidic during their lifetime due, in part, to the foods they eat. The amount of overly acidic foods con-sumed each day in the United States is staggering, especially when you consider that a person needs a slightly alkaline pH to be able to perform to their best and remain in optimal health.

For example, soft drinks such as colas are extremely acidic and create much stress on our pH regulating system. While colas are an unhealthy synthetic creation, there are many popular natural foods that we eat that have pH's that are similar to or even lower than cola drinks, including limes, lemons, orange juice, most berries, cranberry sauce, vinegar, dill and sweet pickles, jams and jellies, and wine.

If you have an overly acidic constitution, the constant consumption of highly acidic food will increase your susceptible to respiratory and other infections. Without understanding the pH content of many foods, you will wonder why you are frequently experiencing symptoms like nasal congestion, sinusitis, sore throats and coughing.

As you look at the chart showing the pH values of common foods and beverages, you will probably be surprised at how many commonly eaten foods are highly acidic. Examples of the various acids contained within our daily fare include acetic acid, which gives vinegar its tartness, and citric acid, found in oranges, lemons, and limes.

Carbonated soft drinks bubble because they are infused with carbon dioxide, a highly acidic substance that is actually a waste product of our own metabolism. A major component of tea is tannic acid. Caffeinated coffee contains many volatile acids, which are particularly abundant in gourmet blends and provide coffee with its desirable rich flavor. Red meat, dairy products, and soft drinks are also high in acidic minerals like sulfur and phosphorus (which are converted to sulfuric acid and phosphoric acid).

Many of these foods are not necessarily "bad." For example, citrus fruits contain vitamin C in the juice and bioflavonoids, which are beneficial antioxidants, in the pulp. They also contain small amounts of alkaline minerals such as potassium (unlike the juices of the other, more tart citrus fruits like lemon, orange and tangerine juices are actually rich sources of the alkaline mineral potassium, despite their low pH).

Whether acid or alkaline in their pH prior to ingestion, many foods can also generate a tremendous amount of acid within the body once they are eaten. For example, protein-rich foods of animal origin, like red meat and dairy products (milk, butter, cheese, ice cream), or tough plant protein like the gluten contained in wheat, rye, barley, and oats appear to be more alkaline in terms of their pH listing in the food chart.

Yet, once they are ingested, they can stimulate the stomach to produce large amounts of hydrochloric acid, which is needed to begin the breakdown of these proteins. These foods also tend to be more inflammatory which can reduce your resistance to respiratory infections. In addition, coffee, alcohol, and fast foods like pizza can also trigger significant hydrochloric-acid production. This increases the acid load within the body that must be buffered.

Wheat and Dairy Products are Mucous Forming

Wheat and dairy products, in particular, tend to be very mucous forming. They can aggravate colds, flus, sinusitis, middle ear infections and bronchitis and should be avoided by people who have repeated respiratory infections. This is not age specific; it is a major issue for many babies, infants, children and adults who are prone to respiratory infections.

Jerry, the husband of my patient, Rachel, would always escort her to her office visits with me and sit in the waiting area. Jerry was a very friendly and high energy person and we would always spend a few minutes visiting. He seemed to enjoy ice cream a great deal and frequently would be eating an ice cream cone.

One day, he and I struck up a conversation and he mentioned that he suffered from frequent earaches as well as sinus congestion. I asked him about his intake of dairy products. He mentioned that he loved ice cream (which was obvious since he was eating an ice cream cone). He also said that he would drink a quart of milk each day.

I suggested that he consider eliminating dairy products and replace them with substitutes like rice milk, and that it might help his respiratory conditions. The next time I saw Jerry, he told me that he had cut out dairy products completely from his diet and that his earaches and sinus conditions were totally gone!

My patient, Samantha, told me that her five-year-old daughter, Tammie, was suffering from frequent ear infections. She recently had a very painful perforated eardrum and was also suffering from digestive upset. She was quite concerned about her daughter and wasn't sure what to do.

After discussing Tammie's diet, I suspected that her wheat and dairy intake were the culprits. I recommended that she eliminate these foods from her diet and instead give her the many wonderful substitutes that are readily available in health food stores and in many supermarkets. After eliminating these foods, Tammie's ear infections decreased significantly and her digestive symptoms eased up, too.

Breast Feeding for Infant's Immunity

As I mentioned earlier in this book, Studies have shown that breast-fed human infants have better resistance to a variety of diseases, including respiratory illnesses, than bottle-fed ones. This is due, in part, to its being a rich source of colostrum. Colostrum is the first milk produced by all mammals after delivery of the newborn. While maternal milk provides important nutrients that are needed for growth and development, colostrum is crucial to the newborn's health since it enhances immunity.

This is because colostrum contains cytokines and other low molecular weight protein compounds that act as biologic response modulators. These substances have profound anti-inflammatory and immunity-enhancing effects.

In one study published in the *British Medical Journal*, samples of human colostrum were examined and all contained respiratory virus neutralizing benefits. Immunoglobulin IgA was found in 18 out of 21 samples. IgA is known to confer protection against upper respiratory infections. This same study also found that breastfeeding conferred significant protection against respiratory illness in infants. Far fewer breast fed infants were admitted to a hospital with severe respiratory illness versus non breast fed infants.

In another research study published in *Pediatrics*, infants in Bangladesh were followed from birth to twelve months of age. Exclusive breastfeeding in these infants was found to confer significant protection against death from acute respiratory illnesses as well as death from diarrhea.

This enhanced immunity is one reason why breastfeeding is so beneficial for infants. I recommend that every mother breastfeed her child until at least one year of age, if at all possible. I have seen a number of infants below the age of a year and a half with frequent respiratory infections. Often, these infants have been fed commercial formulas instead of breast milk, either from birth or because the mother discontinued breastfeeding after a month or two.

How to Modify Common Acidic Foods and Dishes

I have included the following tips to enable you to still enjoy some of the highly acidic but nutritious foods that you may currently be eating. While high-alkaline producers can eat these foods as a regular part of their diet, overly acidic individuals cannot without potentially impairing their immunity and increasing their susceptibility to colds, flus, and lung infections.

Fruit Drinks. Many overly acidic people would like to enjoy blenderized fruit drinks and smoothies because of their delicious taste and high nutrient content. Unfortunately, the high level of acidity of many fruits can cause canker sores, heartburn, abdominal discomfort, and even a drop in energy in overly acidic people.

To neutralize the acidity of the fruit, I recommend using a product called Acid Check, which is gradually released into your body. It is an alkaline mixture containing potassium, magnesium, and calcium that is available in granular and caplet form. I recommend 2 to 3 caplets per day or if you prefer granules mix 1/4 teaspoon into 4-8 ounces of water two times a day between meals.

The granular form comes in a shaker bottle, so you can also use it on the spot to neutralize highly acidic foods such as tomatoes, citrus fruits and juices, berries, salad dressings, spicy foods, sugary foods, and wine. The granules do not alter the flavor or aroma of foods or beverages, but it may make foods taste a little sweeter due to the reduced acid content. Consider keeping a bottle with you for restaurant meals, special occasions, and other times when you don't have as much control over what you eat and need to reduce the meal acidity by as much as 90%.

I also recommend using two to three caplets per day to promote healthy alkalinization or, if you prefer the granules, mix ¼ teaspoon into 4-8 ounces of water two times a day between meals. You can purchase Acid Check at acidcheck.com.

For best digestibility, blenderized fruit drinks and smoothies should be consumed by themselves on an empty stomach, preferably in the morning. If you wish to add protein powder to this drink, use vegetable protein derived from rice or legumes, which are less acidic than animal protein. In addition, do not consume this drink with a protein-rich meal containing meat or milk, since these proteins require more acid production within the stomach for their digestion.

Wine. Many overly acidic individuals would love to drink an occasional glass of wine but find that it causes heartburn and other digestive symptoms. This is because wine has an acidic pH. The alcohol contained within wine also triggers the production of hydrochloric acid within the stomach. As with the fruit drinks, you can also use Acid Check granules to bring up the pH of the wine and neutralize its acidity.

For special social occasions, you can take sodium bicarbonate (baking soda) or a sodium and potassium bicarbonate mixture right after drinking an alcoholic beverage to blunt its acidic effect on the body.

Bicarbonate can also be used to help neutralize the uncomfortable symptoms of an alcohol-induced hangover.

Coffee and Tea. If you feel you cannot live without your daily cup of coffee or black tea, low-acid versions are available from Coffee Bean and Tea Leaf Company (coffeebean.com)

Sparkling Water. If you are at a bar or restaurant and want to drink mineral water but only bubbling varieties are available, you can get rid of the carbonation by adding a pinch of table salt. This will allow the water to go flat, leaving you with a more alkaline drink.

Salad Dressings. You can substitute Bragg Liquid Aminos for vinegar when making salad dressings. Bragg Liquid Aminos is a delicious flavoring agent that can be purchased in most health food stores. Combine it with olive oil and herbs for a delicious dressing. Alternatively, you can prepare a salad dressing by decreasing the amount of vinegar by half and increasing the amount of water and oil, as well as by adding extra flavoring agents such as herbs.

Marinated Vegetables. Avoid vegetables marinated in vinegar. These are highly acidic and are commonly served in Italian and Spanish restaurants and occasionally in American ones.

Many restaurants offer alternative vegetable appet-izers such as steamed asparagus or artichokes. You can also order small side dishes of whatever cooked vegetables are being served that day.

Salt. Sea vegetables are rich in minerals and can be used to replace the more acidic table salt as a flavoring agent. Sea vegetables are now available in shakers to be used as a condiment in natural-food stores.

7

Enzymes to Reduce the Inflammation Caused by Respiratory Infections

When respiratory tissues are inflamed from infection (or allergy), the result is nasal congestion, sore throat, swollen and painful sinuses, itching and tearing of the eyes, fluid in the middle ears, and excess bronchial secretions that lead to coughing. Unfortunately, while over-the-counter drugs can help to suppress coughs, reduce fever, and dry up nasal congestion, they often produce equally unpleasant side effects such as racing heart, drowsiness, and feeling light-headed or drugged.

One of the most effective ways to suppress respiratory inflammation is by taking supplemental enzymes. These include pancreatic enzymes as well as other natural anti-inflammatory substances such as plant-based digestive enzymes like papain, which is derived from papayas, and bromelain, which is derived from pineapples. There are also other powerful anti-inflammatory substances that can greatly reduce your symptoms of respiratory infections that I share with you in this chapter.

Digestive Enzymes Reduce the Inflammation of Respiratory Infections

Let me begin by discussing what are enzymes and how they can help to reduce the inflammation that accompanies respiratory infections.

Our bodies produce thousands of different enzymes, all catalyzing different chemical reactions that are crucial to health and survival. These reactions regulate functions as diverse as the production of energy, digestion, the repair of cells, and the elimination of waste products. Thus, enzymes allow us to breathe, digest, grow, heal, perceive with our senses, and reproduce.

Enzymes affect chemical reactions in the following manner: An enzyme acts on another substance, called a substrate, grasping, holding, and binding the substrate with other molecules to help trigger a chemical reaction. Enzymes allow these reactions to proceed more efficiently, making it possible for them to occur with less expenditure of energy. Thus, an enzyme is a catalyst. Relative to the substances they are acting on, enzymes are present only in small amounts. Moreover, enzymes are not changed by the biochemical processes that they help to initiate.

Because each enzyme has a unique shape that only fits with a certain substance, the various enzymes have very specific functions. For example, pancreatic enzymes, which are discussed in detail in this chapter, break down very specific types of food and are crucial for healthy digestion and absorption and assimilation of the food that we take in through our diet. They also have very dramatic anti-inflammatory benefits and, thus, can offer significant relief from the symptoms of colds, flus, sinusitis and lung infections as well as many other inflammatory conditions. Let's look at this in more detail.

Pancreatic Enzymes and Inflammation

Besides being critical for our digestive processes, a second important function of pancreatic digestive enzymes is to facilitate recovery from tissue damage or injury, including injury caused by bacteria and viruses to the respiratory system through infection,

All traumatic injuries are characterized by an inflammatory response. Similarly, internal injury to tissues due to such stressors as infectious bacteria and viruses (as well as allergens, and toxins) can also cause inflammation.

Inflammation of an injured area is characterized by swelling, heat, and redness. No matter where the site of the injury, the physical manifestations are the same.

When an area of the body becomes inflamed, the blood vessels and capillaries in the injured area begin to dilate (expand), allowing fluids carrying the body's own healing substances to reach the area quickly.

At the same time, the capillary walls become more permeable, and fluids force their way into the surrounding tissue, causing congestion. Very quickly more fluid and waste accumulate than the area can handle. Helper cells seal off the damaged area, creating fibrin clots made of protein, to prevent the spread of bacteria and toxins to surrounding areas. The result is blockage of the blood and lymph vessels, leading to redness, swelling, heat, pain, and the formation of excess fluids in the tissue (edema).

The inflammatory process is controlled by numerous digestive enzymes, especially the body's own pancreatic protein-digesting (proteolytic) enzymes, which eliminate debris at the injury site and initiate the repair of tissue. These enzymes also break up the fibrin, which is made of protein, so that it can be excreted. Digestive enzymes keep the pathological process from spreading and considerably reduce the duration of the injury by speeding up the healing process. Thus, abundant production of digestive enzymes, as well as the use of supplemental enzymes, can greatly limit the severity and scope of inflammatory diseases like colds, flus, sinusitis, middle ear infections and bronchitis and help the body recover more rapidly.

Unfortunately, excessive levels of stress, unhealthy dietary habits of eating difficult to digest, low nutrient content foods (like fats, sugars, fast foods, refined flour products, caffeine and alcohol among others) and the aging process itself takes their toll on our ability to produce adequate levels of digestive enzymes. This not only results in poor digestive function and digestive complaints, but also a decreased ability to suppress and limit the frequency and severity of respiratory infections.

The Use of Supplemental Digestive Enzymes For The Treatment Of Respiratory Infections

There are a wide variety of plant and animal based digestive enzymes that you can take as supplements in addition to eating an enzyme-rich diet. In this section, I will discuss the two main types of supplemental enzymes available and how to use them for the treatment of respiratory infections. They can be taken by both adults and children. For children, they are often available in powder form to mix into food or drinks.

It is important to remember that, when taken with a meal, supplemental enzymes will tend to be used in the digestive process. When taken between meals, on an empty stomach, the enzymes will instead be used by the body for their anti-inflammatory and cellular repair capabilities. For those individuals who have both weak digestive function and other health conditions, the use of supplemental enzymes both with and apart from meals may be most appropriate.

Various types of supplemental enzymes can be combined and taken simultaneously. Many commercial preparations are, in fact, combinations of various enzymes. For example, you may take pancreatic enzymes, bromelain, and papain at the same time to enhance their therapeutic benefits with no adverse effects.

When you are customizing your program, it is helpful to know if your constitution tends to be more alkaline or more acidic. As I mentioned in chapter 3, most people in the United States are overly acidic. Many of these individuals have low production of pancreatic enzymes. If you are overly acidic and enzyme deficient, avoid enzyme products that contain betaine or glutamic hydrochloric acid (HCl) as they may cause a burning sensation in the stomach or increase a tendency toward over acidity. If, on the other hand, you are one of the small number of individuals who have exceedingly good buffering capability, HCl supplementation combined with enzyme products may be beneficial.

Plant-Based Digestive-Enzyme Supplements

I often recommend that my patients who have respiratory infections use supplemental plant-based digestive enzymes as part of their treatment program along with antimicrobial agents and alkalinizing agents. The most readily available plant-based supplemental enzymes are bromelain and papain, which are sold in natural-food stores and pharmacies.

These enzymes supplement those normally made by the stomach and pancreas. Like the digestive enzymes produced within our bodies, they help in the digestion of starches, protein, and fats as well as powerfully suppress the inflammation caused by respiratory and other infections.

Bromelain

Bromelain refers to a family of enzymes extracted from the stem of the pineapple. It has been used over the centuries as a medicinal plant in tropical native cultures around the world and was isolated chemically over 100 years ago. In 1957, bromelain was introduced as a powerful therapeutic compound, used to aid protein digestion and reduce inflammation. Since then, hundreds of scientific papers on its therapeutic applications have been published in the medical literature, ranging from treatment of the common cold to treatment of cancer.

Bromelain and inflammation. Bromelain is a powerful anti-inflammatory substance without the side effects commonly seen with anti-inflammatory medication likes aspirin and other nonsteroidal anti-inflammatory drugs (NSAIDs) such as Ibuprofen (Motrin). These types of drugs account for approximately 100 million prescriptions per year. Tens of millions of individuals also purchase anti-inflammatory medications over the counter, without a doctor's prescription.

Aspirin and these other medications are often used to suppress the inflammatory symptoms of respiratory infections. While these medications are useful in reducing the symptoms of inflammation by suppressing the production of all prostaglandins, they also suppress the beneficial anti-inflammatory ones. In addition, they have no effect on dissolving fibrin clots. Furthermore, long-term use of NSAIDs can lead to liver, kidney, and gastrointestinal side effects.

Unlike NSAIDs, bromelain acts as a natural aspirin without any of the undesirable side effects. Bromelain reduces inflammation in several ways. While aspirin inhibits the synthesis of all prostaglandins (hormone-like chemicals produced within the intestinal tract, uterus, and other sites of the body), bromelain inhibits only the inflammatory ones, without affecting the anti-inflammatory ones.

Bromelain also interacts with fibrin, a tough, clot-like material made of protein that the body manufactures to seal off an injured area. When there is injury, caused by anything from a respiratory infection to a sports accident, the blood vessels and capillaries in the injured area begin to dilate (expand) so the body's own healing substances can reach the area quickly.

At the same time, fluids force their way into the surrounding tissue, causing congestion and resulting in pressure, swelling, heat, and pain. Helper cells then begin to seal off the damaged area, creating fibrin clots made of protein. In an effort to prevent the spread of bacteria and toxins generated by the injury, the fibrin also blocks blood and lymph vessels, which causes more swelling, a blockage of blood flow, and inflammation. The enzymes contained within bromelain help to reduce inflammation by digesting the fibrin clots.

In addition, supplemental bromelain helps to increase the oxygen level in injured tissue and stimulates the body's own natural enzymatic activity without suppressing the immune system, further accelerating the healing process.

Bromelain and respiratory tract infections. Nasal congestion due to respiratory-tract infections is a nuisance, hampering almost any activity. There is scientific evidence that bromelain can be very useful in the treatment of upper-respiratory problems that generate mucus. Bromelain decreases the volume and viscosity of mucus so that it can be more easily cleared from the respiratory tract.

This was shown in a study appearing in *Drugs Under Experimental and Clinical Research*. Volunteers included seventy men and fifty-four women, aged 35 to 75, hospitalized with lung diseases such as chronic bronchitis, pneumonia, and pulmonary abscess.

Patients were randomly given one of three therapies: amoxicillin plus 80 mg of bromelain, amoxicillin plus indomethacin, or amoxicillin alone, every eight hours, for at least eight days or as needed. The sputum (substance expelled by coughing or clearing the throat) of the patients was then analyzed for viscosity. The results of this study showed that bromelain significantly increased the fluidity of mucus. There was also evidence that bromelain combined with drug therapy enhanced the absorption of the amoxicillin.

Children can also benefit from the use of bromelain. The University of Michigan Health System notes that bromelain can be used in children to help treat sinusitis and reduce the symptoms of asthma. A research study published in the journal *In Vivo* found that children with acute sinusitis who were treated with bromelain recovered much more quickly than children treated with medications such as antihistamines, analgesics, and antibiotics or medication and bromelain given together.

The University of Pittsburgh Medical Center also recommends the use of bromelain for digestive problems. This is important since respiratory and digestive symptoms often coexist in children and bromelain can be useful for the treatment of both!

Using bromelain with antibiotics. Several studies in the scientific literature document the effectiveness of bromelain in enhancing the action of antibiotics. In one research study, published in *Experimental Medicine & Surgery*, fifty-three hospitalized patients were given combined antibiotic and bromelain therapy to treat such potentially life-threatening diseases as pneumonia, bronchitis, thrombophlebitis, pyelonephritis, and rectal abscesses. Twenty-three of these patients had been unsuccessfully treated with antibiotic therapy alone. Of these, 22 responded favorably to the combined therapy.

Researchers also compared the length of stay for patients taking antibiotics alone or the combined therapy. Patients with pneumonia or bronchitis who were treated with antibiotics alone remained in the hospital for an average of ten days, as compared with those who also received enzyme therapy, who were able to leave the hospital after only six days.

Another study, published in the journal *Headache*, looked at the use of bromelain in combination with antibiotics for the treatment of acute sinusitis. Forty-eight patients were placed on standard therapy, which included antihistamines and analgesic agents, along with antibiotics, if indicated. Twenty-three patients received bromelain four times daily, while the remaining twenty-five received a placebo. Of the patients receiving bromelain, 87 percent had complete resolution of nasal mucosal inflammation, compared with only 52 percent in the placebo group.

The next time you come down with an acute respiratory infection and your doctor writes you a prescription for antibiotics, be sure to supplement that medication with bromelain. Along with rest, supplementing with bromelain will help you return to your usual activities much more quickly.

Suggested Dosage: Bromelain supplements, in standard dosages of 500 mg taken two to four times per day. Take apart from meals on an empty stomach for best results. It should be combined with bioflavonoids and vitamin C, as these enhance the action of bromelain. Recommended dosages are 500 to 1000 mg of bioflavonoids taken three times a day, and 1000 mg of mineral buffered (alkaline) vitamin C taken two or three times a day apart from meals.

For children, the German Commission E, considered the "gold standard" of evaluating natural herbal medicines, recommends 80 mg to 320 mg of bromelain two to three times a day. It is always advisable to start with the lower doses and see how your child tolerates this supplement. Bromelain may also help to reduce asthma symptoms in children

Factors That Can Inactivate Bromelain. Certain metallic compounds are known to render bromelain inactive, including copper and iron, which are found naturally in many foods, and the heavy metals lead, mercury, and cadmium, which are sometimes present as toxic pollutants in fish and other foods. Heavy-metal contamination can also be found in poor-quality, commercial-grade foods. Buying the highest quality organically grown foods will help you to avoid these enzyme inhibitors.

When shopping for a bromelain supplement, avoid those that combine the bromelain with copper or iron in the same tablet or capsule. Look for bromelain combined with magnesium or cysteine, bromelain activators that enhance its therapeutic effect. The quality of bromelain is expressed in gelatin-digesting units (g.d.u.); the higher the g.d.u., the higher the grade of bromelain and its activity. Keep in mind that bromelain is not heat stable, so supplements need to be stored in a cool place.

Papain. Papain is the enzyme derived from papayas. Best known as a meat tenderizer, it can also be used as a powerful digestant of protein either by itself or combined with bromelain and other digestive enzymes. Research has found that papain has many other clinical applications such as aiding in recovery from injuries and surgery and treating a number of inflammatory conditions such as gluten intolerance.

Along with bromelain, papain is also useful in the treatment of inflammatory conditions that affect our cells and tissues, such as respiratory infections like colds, flus, bronchitis, as well as other inflammatory conditions like arthritis, and thyroiditis. Papain may be beneficial in reducing symptoms of sore throat.

One study, published in *Drugs Under Experimental and Clinical Research*, examined the therapeutic effect of a plant-based digestive enzyme product used in combination with an antibiotic on patients with respiratory illnesses such as chronic bronchitis and pneumonia. The addition of the digestive enzyme to the treatment regimen improved the absorption of the antibiotics and increased their level in the lungs, thereby improving the efficacy of the antibiotics.

In addition, more of the patients on enzyme therapy had total resolution of their symptoms. There were also far fewer patients who failed to respond to the combined therapy than to drug treatment alone.

Enzyme therapy was also found both to reduce the inflammation of the respiratory tissue and to help suppress coughing. In a clinical study involving patients with chronic bronchitis, reduction of coughing was noted after ten days of enzyme therapy. Another research study found that eighty-seven percent of patients undergoing treatment for sinusitis with digestive-enzyme therapy had a significant reduction of their symptoms.

I have seen similar results in my own practice, with many patients experiencing dramatic relief from long-standing sinus conditions after using supplemental digestive enzymes.

Suggested Dosage: 200 to 300 mg of papain with or immediately following meals, upon rising, and before bedtime. The dosage for children has not been established.

Side Effects of Plant Enzymes. While plant enzymes are not known to cause any serious side effects, they may cause increased intestinal gas. Gradually increasing your dosage can improve your tolerance and reduce the likelihood of gas. Plant enzymes should be avoided, as should most supplements, by pregnant women and people with any kind of bleeding disorder.

Plant Based Digestive Enzyme Product

There are a number of excellent digestive enzyme support products available in health food stores and on the Internet. The best products contain blends of plant-based digestive enzymes that target every component of your meals so that your body can break down hard-to-eat foods without gas, bloating, and discomfort. The benefits include:

- Relieves discomfort from gas and bloating
- Breaks down problem foods, including carbohydrates, proteins, fats, starches, and glucose
- Supports optimal intestinal health and function
- Improves nutrient absorption

Plant Based Enzyme Products for Children

There are a number of plant based digestive enzyme products for children that can be taken as a chewable tablet. They are also available for children in powder form that can be into food, drinks, or water. The capsules can also be broken open and sprinkled on food or water. When taken right before eating, many of these products help to support healthy digestion. When taken apart from meals, they can be very useful in reducing the inflammation and symptoms of respiratory infections. These products are widely available in health food stores, the Internet and through Amazon.com. Products include Buddy Bear Digestive Enzymes by Renew Life, BioCor Kids, Enzymedica Kids Digest as well as many other products.

Pancreatic Enzymes Derived from Animal Sources

Although commercial preparations of supplemental pancreatic enzymes are actually derived from the pancreas of animals, particularly cows and pigs, these enzymes are similar to those found in the human body. Pancreatic-enzyme products are unique because they are able to break down all three basic food substances found in our diets: carbohydrates, proteins, and fats. In other words, they contain protein digesting (proteolytic), fat digesting (lipolytic), and starch and sugar digesting (glycolytic) capability.

Pancreatic enzymes, whether produced within the body or taken as supplements, are necessary for normal digestive function. They are also powerful anti-inflammatory and anticlotting agents. Their action occurs at the tissue level in various parts of the body, including muscle and epidermal (skin) tissue. Supplemental pancreatic enzymes can also improve digestion, reducing the workload on the body's own pancreatic enzymes, and facilitate healing from colds, flus, sinusitis, middle ear infections and bronchitis. It is very beneficial to combine them with plant-based enzymes when recovering from a respiratory infection.

I have found pancreatic enzymes to powerfully relieve the inflammatory symptoms of colds, flus, sinusitis, middle ear infections, and bronchitis and consider them to be a mainstay for an effective program to both relieve and prevent these conditions.

How to use pancreatic enzymes

Pancreatic-enzyme products are available in natural-food stores and are sold as tablets or capsules that can vary greatly in size of dose and potency. The potency is indicated by a notation on the label, which is usually a number followed by an X, for instance, 4X or 10X. These have been strictly defined by the United States Pharmacopoeia (USP).

In a 1X pancreatic-enzyme product (pancreatin), each milligram must contain at least 25 USP units of amylase activity, at least 25 USP units of protease activity, and at least 2.0 USP units of lipase activity. Any pancreatic enzyme of higher potency is noted with a whole number greater than 1 to indicate the degree of its greater strength.

For example, a pancreatic extract, full-strength and undiluted, that is eight times stronger than the USP standard would be labeled 8X USP. Full-strength products are generally preferred, as lower-potency pancreatic products may be diluted with substances such as lactose, galactose, and salt.

Pancreatic enzymes are dispensed as powders, capsules, granules, and tablets, the last two available in enteric-coated forms (this means that they don't break down in the stomach). Pancreatic-enzyme supplements with enteric coating may have an advantage because the protective coating allows the pH-sensitive enzymes to pass through the hostile acidic environment of the stomach without being destroyed. Enteric-coated tablets are more likely to reach the small intestine intact, where they are normally used by the body to assist in the breakdown and digestion of foods.

Suggested Dosage: A standard dosage of pancreatic enzymes is one to two tablets, taken with meals if they are meant to be used as a digestive aid. Follow the instructions on the bottle. If a stronger treatment is needed, buy a more potent enzyme product. One of my favorite pancreatic enzyme products is Mega-Zyme. It is a maximum strength product that also contains plant enzymes. It is available through Amazon.com.

If pancreatic enzymes are used to treat inflammatory diseases such as colds, flus, sinusitis, middle ear infections and bronchitis, an accepted dosage is 300 to 1000 mg of high-potency pancreatic enzymes, taken three to four times a day, apart from meals.

When pancreatic enzymes are used in this manner, the supplements need to be taken four times a day, because the enzymes are only active in the body for a maximum of five hours.

It is essential that pancreatic enzymes be taken when the stomach is empty, preferably one-half to one hour before meals, because a considerable amount of the enzymes ability to digest protein is lost in the acid environment of the stomach.

Some enzyme products are enteric-coated, that is, buffered by chemicals like sodium bicarbonate so they will not be attacked by gastric acid or pepsin in the stomach. (See chapters 1 and 2 for a discussion of the dynamics of buffering and pH control.) However, numerous studies have found these to be no more effective, and in some cases, less effective, than uncoated enzymes.

Side effects of pancreatic enzymes

It is well documented in scientific studies that pancreatic enzymes are remarkably free of side effects. However, an excess dosage of these enzymes may cause diarrhea, especially in older patients, and bowel tolerance needs to be monitored. The need for these enzymes diminishes as health returns, and dosages can then be slowly decreased.

A helpful recovery strategy to benefit from digestive enzymes

Deborah and Jeff are two people that I know with very strong immunity who have described to me their amazingly quick recovery from colds, runny noses, and sore throats during the past year. At the first signs of a cold or flu, they leave the office and go home to take a rest or nap and eat lightly and go to bed early. They are normally able to resolve their symptoms rapidly and without the use of drugs and be back at the top of their game in one to two days rather than the two to six weeks that many other people require.

Their instinctive, and obviously successful, strategy in dealing with these minor illnesses plays to their innate strength. These are people with very healthy digestive function who have good digestive enzyme production. They allow the digestive enzymes that they both abundantly produce to reduce the signs of respiratory inflammation.

By immediately reducing their food intake, they can use their digestive enzymes to reduce inflammation instead of to digest a rich meal. These individuals also tend to be naturally alkaline; therefore, they have excellent buffering capability and are able to neutralize the excess acidity seen with infection and allergies, and their strong immune systems are able to overcome any exposure to bacteria or viruses.

If you have weaker digestive function and tend to produce low levels of pancreatic enzymes and are prone to colds, flus, sinusitis, middle-ear infections, and bronchitis, it is very helpful to use supplemental digestive enzymes at the first sign of any of these conditions.

To get the most benefit from these powerful anti-inflammatory enzymes, eat lightly for the first twelve to forty-eight hours after the onset of symptoms, mostly soups and steamed vegetables. In addition, be sure to reduce your level of activity and rest or nap. Finally, consume large amounts of water.

These measures should help to significantly reduce your symptoms in one to two days. In addition, improving your acid/alkaline balance, promoting healthy detoxification, and following a program to increase the oxygen levels within your cells and tissues will help to improve your resistance to respiratory conditions.

If you are prone to respiratory conditions and tend to travel frequently, or are involved in stressful work or recreational activities, be sure to always have an emergency kit with you that contains supplemental digestive enzymes as well as the cold remedies described in this book, such as sodium and potassium bicarbonate, colloidal silver, and anti-inflammatory and anti-infectious herbs such as echinacea and ginger.

Other Anti-Inflammatory Supplements That Benefit Respiratory Illnesses

Besides digestive enzymes there are a number of other nutritional supplements that are beneficial for reducing the inflammation that occurs with respiratory illnesses. I describe some of the most useful ones in this section.

Turmeric

Turmeric has been used for thousands of years in Indian cooking and in India's traditional Ayurvedic medicine. The turmeric plant, grown from India to Indonesia, is related to ginger and has pulpy, orange, tuberous roots that grow to about two feet in length. It is an indispensable part of the mixture of spices known as curry powder. The medicinally active compound in turmeric is curcumin, the rich orange-yellow pigment that gives turmeric its characteristic orange-yellow color.

For thousands of years, curcumin has been used in both Chinese and Indian systems of medicine as an anti-inflammatory agent and for the treatment of numerous health conditions. Modern research corroborates its use as an anti-inflammatory. Turmeric is very effective when used for the treatments of respiratory infections and helps to reduce the redness and swelling that usually accompanies infections of the sinuses, throat and chest.

In one interesting research study, curcumin was even found to be as effective as cortisone, a potent medical anti-inflammatory. This article noted that an added benefit of curcumin is that it does not normally cause side effects, providing a safe alternative to these powerful anti-inflammatory drugs, which can cause gastric irritation and even peptic ulcers in susceptible people.

Curcumin's therapeutic benefits occur through several mechanisms. Curcumin reduces inflammation by inhibiting leukotriene formation and platelet aggregation. It also promotes the breakup of blood clots and inhibits the inflammatory response to various stimuli. There is some indication that curcumin has an indirect effect on reducing inflammation through the adrenal gland or its hormones.

The most likely explanation is that it increases the effectiveness of the body's own cortisone, one of the body's major anti-inflammatory hormones. Curcumin may do this by sensitizing or priming cortisone receptor sites, thereby potentiating cortisone's action. It may also act by increasing the half-life of cortisone through reducing its breakdown by the liver. While the long-term use of prescription cortisone has been associated with serious side effects, including adrenal atrophy, osteoporosis, and diabetes mellitus, curcumin has been found to be as effective as cortisone with no toxicity.

Suggested Dosage: The recommended dosage for curcumin as an anti-inflammatory agent is 400 to 600 mg three times a day. It is often formulated with an equal amount of bromelain to enhance absorption. This combination is best taken on an empty stomach, twenty minutes before meals or between meals. Toxicity reactions have not been reported at standard dosage levels. The dosage for infants and small children should not exceed ½ teaspoon as a warm tea or the liquid mixed with food each day for the relief of nasal and chest congestion, not to be taken more than three days.

Since curcumin has blood-thinning effects, its use should be avoided in people on blood thinning drugs like Coumadin. It should not be used by pregnant or nursing women.

Ginger

Ginger is a pungent, spicy herb native to southern Asia. For thousands of years, ginger has been an important herb used in traditional Asian medicine. It is now cultivated throughout the tropics in countries as diverse as Jamaica, India, and China. It is used as a spice in many cuisines and as a flavoring agent for beverages such as ginger ale and in many baked goods.

Ginger is a powerful anti-inflammatory agent. It works through modulating or balancing the prostaglandin pathway. Chemicals in ginger have been found to inhibit inflammatory chemicals like thromboxanes and leukotrienes, which have been linked to conditions like asthma and coronary-artery spasm. On the other hand, these chemicals do not interfere with the production of beneficial anti-inflammatory prostaglandins. As a result, ginger has been found to reduce inflammation, pain, and fever in a variety of conditions including colds, flus, sinusitis and lung infections. As such, its effects are similar to medications like aspirin, without the toxic side effects.

Suggested Dosage: Dry, powdered ginger root can be used in dosages of 500 to 1000 mg per day.

Tripling or quadrupling this dosage may provide more rapid relief. However, dosages should not be used beyond this level.

Ginger root should not be given to children under 2 years of age, according to the University of Maryland Medical Center. Older children can use ginger, but in dosages lower than those recommended for adults. A child weighing 100 pounds can take one half of the lowest dose used by adults. A child weighing 50 pounds can be given one-third of the lowest adult dose.

I particularly like the use of ginger tea when recovering from respiratory infections and have found it to be very helpful. Mix 1/2 tsp. ground ginger or 1 to 2 tsp. grated fresh ginger with 1 tsp. honey. Add one cup of boiling water to make a cup of ginger tea. You can also make a pot of brewed ginger tea and sip on it throughout the day. I recommend 2-3 tbsp of chopped ginger added to 5 cups boiling water. Let simmer for 20 minutes.

Licorice Root

The use of licorice has a long history, appearing prominently in the first great Chinese herbal The Pen Tsao Ching (Classic of Herbs), written more than 5000 years ago. Licorice today is one of the most prescribed herbs in the Chinese pharmacopoeia, second only to ginseng. Licorice has also long been used in the West for medicinal purposes. Bundles of licorice were found amid the treasures of King Tut's tomb, and licorice appears in European herbals (an herbal is a book about plants) from the Renaissance to modern times, usually prescribed and referenced as a diuretic.

The primary active component in licorice is glycyrrhizin, which has a broad range of benefits. The licorice root is fifty times sweeter than sugar. In studies, licorice has been used effectively to control hepatitis and improve liver function in people with cirrhosis.

Contemporary herbalists recommend licorice for its soothing effects on respiratory and gastrointestinal tracts because of its anti-inflammatory properties. Licorice tea is very helpful when fighting off a cold. In a study published in *The Lancet*, fifty patients with gastric ulcers were successfully treated with licorice, which was as effective as treatment with a drug such as cimetidine.

Licorice also stimulates cell production of interferon, the body's own antiviral compound. In an animal study done at the University of Texas, the test subjects were exposed to high doses of the influenza virus. Half of the animals were given glycyrrhizin, which is the active ingredient found in licorice, a day before being infected with the flu virus as well on days one and four following exposure to the virus. The other half of the animals were treated as a placebo group and only given saline injections.

After three weeks, all of the treated animals were still alive while all animals given only the placebo had died. The mechanism of action for this beneficial effect from the licorice extract was found to be the stimulation of the production of interferon. Licorice can also be used in nutritional programs to treat bacterial and fungal infections.

Suggested Dosage: Licorice is included in the FDA's list of herbs generally regarded as safe. Overdose reports have involved highly concentrated licorice extracts used in some candies, laxatives, and tobacco products. I love licorice tea for its delicious sweetness.

To take licorice as a tea, gently boil 1/2 tsp. of the powdered herb in one cup of water for ten minutes. Drink up to two cups a day.

Children with body weights of 50 lb. or more can drink 1/3 a cup of licorice tea three times a day for relief of sore throats treatment. Licorice tea should not be given to children who weigh less than 50 lb. or to infants.

Licorice root is also available in 300 mg capsules; take one capsule between meals two times per day.

However, licorice should not be used by pregnant and nursing women. Long-term use of licorice, more than four weeks, should be avoided by anyone with a history of diabetes, glaucoma, high blood pressure, stroke, or heart disease, as licorice can cause water retention and a rise in blood pressure.

8

Cold and Flu-Like Symptoms due to Impaired Detoxification

Cold, flus and lung infections are also much more common when our detoxification capacity is impaired. Detoxification is one of our body's most crucial physiological functions. It refers to the process of neutralizing or transforming substances that would normally be poisonous or harmful, and eliminating them from the body. Without proper detoxification, toxic substances would accumulate within the body and impair our health by interfering with the function of all our vital organ systems.

Good detoxification is a major factor in preventing illnesses. It prevents toxic chemicals from accumulating in the body, which can cause a wide variety of distressing symptoms such as brain fog, aching joints and muscles, digestive symptoms. It is also the first line of protection against the development of cold, flu, lung infections and other infectious disease

The Liver – Our Primary Organ of Detoxification

The liver is our primary organ of detoxification. It is the main interface between both ingested and internally created toxins and all the cells of our bodies. If the liver can handle the toxic load we put on our bodies, we can perform at our best and remain healthy. However, if liver function is impaired, our health is negatively affected and we are much more prone towards cold and flus.

The liver is one of the most complex and metabolically active organs in the body. It is also the largest organ in the body (aside from the skin), normally weighing about four pounds. The liver lies in the upper right portion of the abdominal cavity beneath the diaphragm. Its large size reflects the multiple functions it performs. It carries out hundreds, if not thousands, of enzymatic reactions along numerous metabolic pathways, playing a pivotal role in maintaining health.

The liver is so crucial to health that it is the only organ that can completely regenerate itself when part of it is removed or damaged. Up to 25 percent of the liver can be removed, and it can still perform its tasks. Moreover, its powers of regeneration are awesome: Within a short period of time, the liver will grow back to its original shape and size.

As harmful chemicals and bacteria circulate through the liver, they pass through a network of blood vessels called the portal system. Unlike other organs of the body, the portal system does not receive blood from the heart. Instead, the liver receives much of its blood directly from the intestinal tract. This allows the liver to process the nutrients and any ingested pollutants before they reach the general circulation. The liver processes about three pints of blood, or an average of 29 percent of a person's total cardiac output, per minute.

How the Liver Neutralizes Bacteria, Viruses and Toxins

The liver deactivates and removes the toxic chemicals and harmful bacteria and other pathogens that circulate throughout the body by two methods. The first method consists of filtering viruses and bacteria through channels called sinusoids. The second method consists of an extensive two-step system of enzymes that facilitate the deactivation and elimination of toxins. When functioning optimally, these two systems help to prevent colds, flus and lung infections from occurring.

Method 1: Filtering Viruses and Bacteria

Blood flowing through the intestinal capillaries picks up many bacteria from the intestines. Within the liver, the Kupffer cells line the hepatic sinuses. These cells engulf and digest about 99 percent of the bacteria present. This occurs through a process called phagocytosis, the process in which one molecule digests another. Only the remaining one percent of the bacteria escapes destruction within the liver and is able to pass through the liver into the general circulation.

Bacteria and yeast can also form toxins that are absorbed into the bloodstream and carried throughout the body. These microbes are implicated in various diseases, including ulcerative colitis, thyroid disease, allergies, and immune disorders. The healthy liver filters out these pathogens, further reducing stress on the immune system. When this function is impaired, individuals are much more susceptible to developing recurrent colds, flus and lung infections.

Method 2: Detoxification of Harmful Chemicals

Many potentially toxic chemicals can also impair our immunity and cause cold and flu-like symptoms such as runny nose, sinus congestion and coughing. These chemicals are normally detoxified within the liver through the second method, which consists of an extensive two-step system of enzymes that facilitates the deactivation and elimination of toxins.

Phase I involves a group of enzymes called the cytochrome P-450 system. This system contains between fifty and a hundred enzymes, each of which detoxifies specific types of chemicals. In this phase, toxins undergo oxidation and reduction, in which electrons are transferred between molecules. They are also rendered more water-soluble.

Most harmful chemicals — such as pesticides, herbicides, alcohol, and drugs — are fat soluble when they first enter the body, which allows them to be stored in our fatty tissue and therefore makes them more difficult to eliminate from the body. But when toxins are rendered water soluble, they can be more easily excreted through the kidneys and intestinal tract. Phase I of the detoxification process reduces the toxicity of chemicals that would be harmful to the body if they were allowed to remain in their original state.

After this phase, toxins are either neutralized, excreted from the body through the intestines or urinary tract, or converted into an intermediate form suitable for further processing by the phase II detoxification system. As these intermediate products are formed, free radicals are generated, and antioxidants are necessary to keep these free radicals from damaging the liver.

In phase II of the detoxification process, the intermediate compounds generated in phase I are transformed into harmless metabolites (breakdown products) that can then be excreted by the body. Phase II enzymes act directly on some toxic substances through a process called conjugation, in which these substances are bound with a protective compound. This process either inactivates or neutralizes the toxins or enables them to be more readily eliminated from the body. Conjugated toxins are excreted through the urinary tract or the intestines.

Over the years, I have seen a number of patients develop cold and flulike symptoms when exposed to toxic chemicals like formaldehyde, toluene, or benzene. I have also seen these symptoms in patients whose livers could not handle prescription drugs that were prescribed by their physicians for specific medical purposes. I have seen patients develop a runny nose, sneezing, and even chills when administered a local anesthetic for minor surgery.

I have even seen these types of symptoms after patients ingested synthetic hormones like Synthroid, a replacement therapy for low thyroid function, or Provera, a synthetic form of progesterone, as well as prednisone, an adrenal hormone used to treat many inflammatory conditions.

The cold and flu-like symptoms did not abate in these individuals until they were able to avoid exposure to the environmental toxins that they could not tolerate or until they discontinued the use of the offending drug. Symptoms often continued after minor surgery until the anesthetic was finally detoxified by the body. Prescription drugs are not the only culprits. I have also found that some patients develop nausea, bloating, and other symptoms of poor liver function after taking oil-based nutritional supplements such as vitamin E, evening primrose oil, and certain herbs.

All of these substances must be broken down by the enzyme systems of the liver and then excreted from the body so as not to accumulate to toxic levels. The individuals who suffer from such extreme suscept-ibility to environmental chemicals, medications, and nutrients are unable to detoxify them efficiently due to poor liver function.

The symptoms of colds and flus are quality of life saboteurs, making you feel miserable and often resulting in lost work time. If you frequently suffer from these symptoms, it is important to differentiate between the symptoms caused by infectious disease and reactions that are due to exposure to a toxic substance you cannot tolerate.

While colds and flus need to be treated by suppressing the pathogens and restoring your body's buffering, enzyme, and oxygenation functions, similar types of symptoms due to toxic chemical exposure need to be treated differently. Toxic chemicals need to be detoxified and eliminated from the body through healthy liver function. Remember that cells within the liver also help to destroy disease-causing bacteria.

If you are susceptible to specific drugs or nutrients, their use should be discontinued and further use avoided. However, be sure to consult with your physician before discontinuing any prescription drugs. If your symptoms seem to be due to the use of nutritional supplements, use non-oil-based sub-stitutes. In addition, you should follow a liver restoration program such as the one described next in this chapter to help restore your detoxification capability.

Combatting Colds, Flus and Lung Infections Through the Detoxification Diet

Because our livers tend to get so overworked and stressed, it is important to follow a dietary program that supports the health and function of your liver and even incorporate periodic fasting. This will help to maintain your ability to detoxify efficiently and restore your resistance to cold, flus and bronchitis.

This means eliminating foods that put wear and tear on the liver and stress our bodies such as high fat and sugar laden foods, rich desserts, caffeine, alcohol, fast foods like pizza and cheeseburgers, fried foods, white flour products, and additives. It means eating a diet that is primarily composed of whole, unrefined, high nutrient foods. These foods should be organic, unsprayed and unprocessed, whenever possible. It is essential to follow a dietary program that emphasizes lighter, easier to digest foods as well as foods that are beneficial for the liver's functioning.

I have found that when my patients have followed a diet to support healthy liver function and enhance detoxification, they usually begin to notice a rapid reduction in their physical symptoms of ill health. Besides better resistance to infections and fewer episodes of cold, flus and bronchitis, their level of energy and vitality usually is increased as well as their mental clarity and sharpness. Feelings of emotional stress, like being on an "emotional roller coaster," start to smooth out. The mood becomes more calm and balanced. The liver responds quickly to a lighter, healthier diet, especially if the intake of toxic substances that burden it is significantly reduced. An added benefit is that you may find that you begin to shed unwanted pounds and that chronic health issues begin to improve.

When you are customizing your own liver detox-ification program, it is important to both cleanse the liver and strengthen and restore its functional capacity at the same time. Since powerful reactions such as headaches, fatigue, and even a runny nose can occur with any detoxification program, you must start slowly and gradually work up to suggested levels.

All dietary changes that are made to improve liver function should be done gradually, over several weeks to several months. As with all health progr- ams, you must experiment within known safe ranges to find the levels that work for your individual biochemistry.

I recommend that you eat a vegetarian emphasis diet, with an emphasis on raw foods or lightly steamed foods. Daily meals should incorporate a variety of salads, fresh fruits and vegetables, whole grains, and legumes. These foods, which are made up of simple molecules of starch, cellulose, antioxidants, fruit sugars, and other easy-to-metabolize substances, place minimum stress on the liver.

Some people need a higher intake of protein to maintain their level of energy. If animal protein is desired, small to moderate amounts of easy-to- assimilate fish, free-range poultry and eggs can be added. Oils should be high quality cold-pressed monounsaturated and polyunsaturated vegetable oils — used only in small amounts in the early stages of recovery.

In terms of your main meal of the day, many people on a detoxification diet do well with their plate divided up between ½ vegetables or salad, ¼ complex carbohydrate like whole grains and ¼ protein. This can vary, of course, based on your own individual dietary needs. Breakfast can includes smoothies and nutritious whole grain cereals with ingredients like ground flax meal, which benefit digestion or easily digestible protein based dishes, as needed.

More Specific Information on Diet

Traditional Chinese Medicine recommends the use of certain plant-based foods as part of a dietary regimen for restoring liver function. I have found in my clinical practice that the following foods are well tolerated and seem to accelerate the healing of liver-related problems: beets, broccoli, cabbage, Brussels sprouts, turnips, kale, parsley, lettuce, cucumber, green foods such as spirulina, chlorella, and barley grass, beans and peas, sprouts, tofu, rice, millet, and fresh fruits, preferably consumed during the warmer months.

As previously mentioned previously, the interme-diate products created through the process of detoxification are potentially dangerous, it is important that phase II of detoxification be function-ing properly to be able to complete the metabolism of these toxins. Foods such as broccoli, Brussels sprouts, cabbage, oranges, tangerines, dill, and caraway seeds can support this function. Broccoli, Brussels sprouts, and cabbage contain indole-3-carbinol and oranges, tangerines, dill, and caraway seeds contain limonene, both of which stimulate the phase I detoxification enzymes. However, I recommend avoiding citrus fruits, as well as vinegar, if you tend towards over acidity and respiratory infections.

In contrast, a diet that includes large amounts of red meat, dairy products, and fatty foods like nuts and chips burden the liver, which must break down the large and more complex structures of these proteins and fats into triglycerides, prostaglandins, and an array of waste products that can be excreted by the body. When the liver cannot process fats, they accumulate inside liver cells, creating fatty degeneration of the liver. In time, these fats will be deposited in the arteries, leading to eventual heart problems and stroke.

As previously mentioned, to decrease stress on the liver, it is also critical to avoid certain substances, such as refined white sugar and flour, alcohol, caffeine, and drugs (other than needed prescribed medicines), because the breakdown of these products leaves toxic residues that the liver must neutralize. Following a lighter, fresher diet allows the liver to go through a gradual self-cleansing process, without causing further stress.

Eat only those foods that do not add to the stress load on the liver. Constantly experiment with the suggested food groups and find those you like and tolerate best. Incorporate these foods into recipes you enjoy or find recipes that use these food groups. Remember, it is virtually impossible to rebuild and restore liver function without eliminating foods that are high in fat and sugar content.

Individuals who are following a program to restore their detoxification capability may still want to enjoy an occasional meal of animal protein. The following suggestions will put the least strain on your liver. Eat eggs prepared simply, either soft- or hard-boiled. Avoid eggs prepared with fats and oils such as deviled, fried, or scrambled eggs. Choose soft-textured, easy-to-digest fish such as salmon, trout and other fish rich in healthful omega 3 fatty acids, which reduce inflammation within the body. It is best to avoid red meat such as pork, lamb, or beef, which are high in saturated fat and more fibrous in texture, and therefore more difficult to digest.

While you are restoring your liver function, eliminate all alcoholic beverages. Switch to mineral water and herbal teas such as chamomile and peppermint, which are therapeutic for the liver. Once liver function is restored, alcohol intake should be limited to an occasional, single beverage.

Individuals with impaired detoxification function should make an effort to avoid eating after 6:00 p.m. or 7:00 p.m. at the very latest. In addition, eat your heaviest meals early in the day, with your last meal being the lightest. This will help to prevent undue stress on the liver during the night when it should be repairing and restoring itself rather than trying to metabolize the residues of a heavy meal. Eating late at night can significantly retard a liver restoration program. My patients have found that avoiding heavy meals eaten late at night significantly reduces morning grogginess and brain fog.

All dietary changes that are made to improve liver function should be done gradually, over several weeks to several months. Too extreme and rapid a change in one's diet can induce waste products to be eliminated more rapidly than the liver can handle, triggering symptoms like nasal congestion, flu-like symptoms, diarrhea, bad breath, and aches and pains.

As with a detoxification diet, you can continue taking any nutritional supplements that you would normally use during a modified fast in order to provide your body with the essential support that it needs.

One of my patients, Karen, suffered from frequent colds, chronic sinusitis and fatigue. She had recently lost her job as an administrative assistant and took on a temporary position. To her dismay, it turned out that the office had been recently decorated with new carpeting and furniture, all of which were made from synthetic materials and were releasing toxic fumes. Immediately after beginning the job, these toxins put her immune system over the edge. She began to suffer from brain fog and dizziness as well as a constant runny nose. Recognizing that the chemicals emanating from the new furnishings were probably causing her symptoms, she quit that job immediately and came to me for help.

I recognized that Karen not only needed to boost her immune function and eliminate her tendency towards respiratory infections, but also needed to strengthen her detoxification capacity, as well. Besides my respiratory infection supplement program, I recommended that she begin a detoxification diet to reduce the toxin load on her liver. She also read my book on detoxification, **Dr. Susan Lark's Complete Guide to Detoxification,** since she was very interested in learning about other liver cleansing techniques.

While her exposure to a significant toxin load at her temporary job was the tipping point for Karen, it turned out to be a blessing in disguise. Not only did her brain fog, dizziness and constant runny nose resolve, but her chronic sinusitis and tendency towards frequent colds did as well. She also enjoyed her newly restored energy and vitality!

Modified Fasting

Many books on detoxification recommend fasting as the quickest and most efficient way to rid the body of accumulated toxins, but true fasting is very difficult for the average American. A true fast means consuming only water or diluted liquids such as juices, broths, or herbal teas for a prescribed period of time.

Fasting has been practiced for thousands of years by the people of nearly all cultures all over the world. Used for purification, penance, during periods of mourning, and to strengthen mental, physical, and spiritual powers, fasting is an ancient practice with modern applications.

However, most of us in the United States live busy, stressful lives, with myriad responsibilities at home, school, and work. We don't often have the luxury of a large block of time without responsibilities to undertake the intensity of a true fast.

Fasting can accelerate the elimination of toxins from the body and trigger a number of uncomfortable symptoms including nasal discharge, headache and flu-like symptoms.

If you are working and active, a true fast can be very disruptive. However, I have found with my own patients that many of them do best with a program of two or three light meals a day.

These meals can consist of fruit and vegetable juices; low-sodium and low-fat broths; smoothies; herbal teas; light, easy-to-digest solid foods, such as uncooked or lightly steamed organic vegetables and sprouts; and smaller amounts of thoroughly cooked starches, grains, and legumes. Such a program can be followed for a few days up to several weeks, although some people may choose to do this for an even longer period of time. This program will help to begin to clear toxins from the liver.

You should preferably consume organic fruits, vegetables, grains and legumes during a modified fast, because if you are trying to eliminate toxins from the body, consuming foods covered with chemical pesticides and fertilizers is counterproductive. Fruit and vegetable juices should be prepared fresh, used within a day or two, and always kept refrigerated. Some bottled vegetable juices may be used when fresh ones are unavailable. Excellent vegetable juices include carrot, beet and beet greens, parsley, celery, cucumber, kale and spinach, but a wide variety of other vegetables can be used for juicing. To enhance the cleansing action of these juices, add a little garlic or wheatgrass juice.

However, don't drink fruit juices by themselves because they are highly acidic and high in concentrated sugars. Fruit juices can be mixed with vegetable juices if you miss the sweet flavor of fruit. If you can't live without some fresh fruit juice, the best ones are papaya and melon, preferably diluted by 50 percent with water. But if you are hypoglycemic or suffer from fatigue, you should avoid drinking fruit juice completely. The simple sugars found in fruit juices will cause an overproduction of insulin by the pancreas. This, in turn, will trigger the roller-coaster effect of quick highs and sudden lows in blood sugar levels.

In contrast, eating the whole fruit slows down absorption of the sugar because of the fiber contained within the fruit. In addition, when fruit juices are mixed with protein and oils (like protein powder or ground flaxseed) as is commonly done with smoothies, the sugar from the juice is absorbed much more slowly and does not cause a hypoglycemic type of effect.

Smoothies are great meals to prepare during a detoxification diet or modified fast because they contain the full range of nutrients needed to maintain your level of energy. Yet, they do not put stress on the digestive organs, including the liver, because all of the ingredients are already broken down into small particles and liquefied in a blender, thereby making digestion much easier. I share with you a number of great smoothie recipes in the recipe section of this book that support healthy digestion and detoxification.

You can continue taking any nutritional supplements that you would normally use during a modified fast in order to provide your body with the essential support that it needs.

9

Healthy Oxygenation Helps to
Prevent Colds, Flus and Bronchitis

Oxygen is a clear, odorless gas that easily dissolves in
water. Oxygen is the most important element needed
to sustain life. Humans can survive without food for
many weeks and can go without water for several
days but can only survive without oxygen for a
matter of minutes. As you will learn in this chapter,
having healthy levels of oxygen in the body is
necessary to sustain the energy and vitality of all our
cells and tissues. It is also essential to prevent
respiratory and other infections.

How Oxygen Is Used Within the Body

Oxygen is primarily taken into the body by the lungs
during respiration. We breathe oxygen into our lungs
from the environment, normally inhaling twelve to
twenty times a minute while at rest. It is the primary
fuel that supports all of the biochemical processes
that occur in our tissues and cells. It supplies the
energy for the maintenance, growth, and repair of all
our cells and is crucial for maintaining our health and
well-being.

The oxygen we breathe reacts with glucose (sugar), which is derived from the foods that we eat and from the breakdown of starches and fats in the body. This reaction produces carbon dioxide, water, and energy. The energy that is created from this reaction is stored in the body as adenosine triphosphate (ATP), which is often referred to as the basic energy currency of the body. ATP is needed for all of the tasks that our cells must perform to maintain the health and integrity of the body

Because of its role in energy production, oxygen is essential for the transport of molecules, the synthesis of chemical compounds, and mechanical work like muscle contraction. Hundreds of thousands of these reactions are going on at all times. Because of these reactions, the heart is able to pump blood, the immune system to fight infections, the gastrointestinal tract to digest foods, and the nervous system and brain to process information.

Oxygen is also alkaline and thereby helps the cells to maintain the slightly alkaline pH necessary for optimal health and good immunity. (I discussed the importance of a slightly alkaline pH for immunity and resistance to respiratory illnesses in chapter 2). It also helps to protect us from becoming overly acidic through its role in removing waste products from the body.

When food is broken down and converted into energy, carbon residues can accumulate and must be removed from the body. This carbon combines with oxygen to form carbon dioxide, an acidic waste product of metabolism that is excreted from the body through the lungs.

Thus, when a cell is highly oxygenated, it is able to create energy (ATP), maintain its alkalinity, and sustain an environment that is incompatible with most disease-causing microorganisms. However, when the amount of oxygen in the body is reduced below optimal levels, this creates an environment in the cells that is conducive to the growth of infectious microorganisms such as those that cause colds, flus, sinusitis, middle ear infections and bronchitis.

Most pathogens are anaerobic — that is, they thrive in an environment that is low in oxygen and has an acidic pH. In fact, infectious microorganisms such as bacteria, viruses, fungi, and parasites as well as cancer cells produce their energy (ATP) through the fermentation of glucose instead of through oxygen. These pathogens are unable to survive in a cellular environment that is oxygen rich and slightly alkaline, which is why it is so critically important for the prevention of respiratory infections and optimal health, in general, that we remain highly oxygenated and maintain our pH in a slightly alkaline state.

The Importance of Deep Breathing to Prevent Respiratory Infections

Often, our busy stress filled lives make deep, healthy breathing more difficult. Many of us go through our days in a fast paced way, trying to deal with what seems like an unending stream of small issues on our "to do lists" as well as the big issues that arise in our lives like family problems, financial concerns, illness in family members or friends and a number of other major items.

When you are stressed or tense, breathing becomes more erratic and shallow. This is also true if you are feeling pain or discomfort in your body. When you are feeling pain, breathing tends to become jagged, erratic, and shallow and your oxygen levels decrease. With both of these conditions, you tend to tense and tighten your muscles, constrict blood flow, elevate your pulse rate and heartbeat, and stimulate the output of stressful chemicals from your glands. Waste products such as carbon dioxide and lactic acid also accumulate in your muscles and other tissues.

As a result, your oxygen levels will decrease. You may find yourself breathing too fast, or you may even stop breathing altogether and hold your breath for periods of time without realizing it. This decreases our level of oxygenation. If you are already predisposed towards colds, flus and bronchitis, this can increase your risk of developing respiratory infections even more.

If you catch yourself doing this, it is very beneficial to stop what you are doing and take a "breath break." Taking time each day to relax for a few minutes and do breathing exercises can reverse this pattern of stress and help restore a sense of peace and calm to your life as well as support healthy immunity.

In this section, I share with you several breathing exercises that I have developed to help restore healthy breathing and oxygenation. If you tend to be a shallow breather, I recommend that you practice the on a regular basis. Many of my patients have practiced these exercises along with other stress reduction techniques and have found them to be very helpful.

I recommend that you do these exercises in a slow and relaxed manner. Breathing slowly and deeply allows you take in large amounts of oxygen from the environmental air. Full expansion of the lungs in a relaxed, rhythmic way facilitates maximal oxygen uptake by the body. It is important to allow both the stomach and the rib cage to relax while breathing so that air can fill the entire lungs. This type of breathing strengthens the muscles in the abdomen and chest, relaxes the body, and allows for the most efficient oxygenation.

When you begin your breathing exercise session, it is important to find a comfortable position. You should do some exercises lying on your back; for other exercises, you will be sitting up. Unless otherwise directed, keep your arms and legs uncrossed and your back straight. You can do them in a bright and cheerful part of your home or even outdoors in your backyard or in a park.

Exercise 1: Deep Abdominal Breathing

Deep, slow abdominal breathing is a very important technique to optimize our intake of oxygen, increase our level of energy and bring us a sense of deep inner peace, calm and joy. It helps brings more oxygen, the fuel for metabolic activity, to all tissues of the body. Rapid, shallow breathing decreases oxygen supply and keeps one devitalized. Deep breathing helps to relax the entire body, and strengthens muscles in the chest and abdomen. It also helps calm many other physiological processes, such as rapid pulse rate and heartbeat that often accompany stress and pain.

* Lie flat on your back with your knees pulled up. Keep your feet slightly apart. Try to breathe in and out through your nose.

* Inhale deeply. As you breathe in, allow your stomach to relax so that the air flows into your abdomen. Your stomach should balloon out as you breathe in. Visualize your lungs filling up with air so that your chest swells out.

* Imagine that the air you breathe is filling your body with energy.

* Exhale deeply. As you breathe out, let your stomach and chest collapse. Imagine the air being pushed out, first from your abdomen and then from your lungs.

Exercise 2: Peaceful, Slow Breathing

Breathing slowly and peacefully can actually decrease stress and tension and help to promote a sense of inner calm and quiet. Such breathing helps our mind to slow down and our emotions to be happier and more harmonious. Life feels good. We make better decisions and relate to those around us in a healthier way when we are calm.

Breathing slowly can also calm our physical responses by helping to balance autonomic nervous system function. The autonomic nervous system regulates functions that we are usually not aware of, such as circulation of the blood, muscle tension, pulse rate, breathing, and glandular function.

The autonomic nervous system is divided into two parts that oppose and complement each other, the sympathetic and parasympathetic systems. The sympathetic nervous system is linked to tension and the "fight or flight" response of fear and panic, while the parasympathetic nervous system regulates body responses that are relaxed and calm.

Slow, peaceful breathing is a way to calm down these stress responses and bring the body back to a state of balance. By slowing down our breathing, we slow down our other physiologic responses. Our muscles relax and our blood vessels dilate; a state of equilibrium is restored.

- Lie flat on your back with your knees pulled up. Keep your feet slightly apart. Try to breathe in and out through your nose.

- Inhale deeply. As you breathe in, allow your stomach to relax so that the air flows into your abdomen. Let your stomach balloon out as you breathe in. Visualize the lowest parts of your lungs filling up with air.

- Imagine that the air you are breathing in is filled with peace and calm. A sensation of peacefulness and calm is filling every cell of your body. Your whole body feels warm and relaxed as you breathe in this air. Now, exhale deeply. As you breathe out, imagine the air being pushed out from the bottom of your lungs to the top.

- Repeat this sequence until your entire body feels relaxed and your breathing is slow and regular.

Exercise 3: Muscle Tension Release Breathing

This exercise will help you to get in touch with and release general muscle tension and tightness. Often we carry extra tension in our bodies when we are feeling stressed, driving in rush hour traffic, dealing with upset children, doing intense deskwork or even competitive sports. These are typical of activities that may cause us to tense our muscles and breathe less deeply. We may unconsciously tense up muscles throughout the entire body. Doing intense work at the computer frequently also creates tension in the neck, shoulders.

This exercise will help you focus on any tension that you are carrying in your upper body. As you relax and release the muscles in your neck and shoulders, it will help to release muscle tension in your entire body. This is a good exercise to do while walking or doing sports or deskwork, to get in touch with any muscle tension that you may be carrying.

- Sit upright in a chair. Be sure you are in a comfortable position. Keep your feet slightly apart. Try to breathe in and out through your nose.

- Inhale and exhale deeply. As you breathe, let your head move from side to side, keeping your shoulders down. As you do this movement, imagine that your neck is made out of putty and that it allows your head to move in a supple, relaxed movement from the left to the right.

- Now inhale and pull your shoulders up towards your ears.

- Hold your breath and keep your shoulders in a hunched position. Exhale and let your shoulders drop back into a relaxed, comfortable position. Repeat this several times.

- Inhale and exhale deeply as you roll your shoulders forward. Make a large, slow, circular motion with your shoulders. Then, roll your shoulders back slowly. Repeat this several times.

- Inhale and exhale deeply, keeping the rest of your body still and relaxed. Repeat this several times.

Exercise 4: Emotional Cleansing Breath

I have seen, during my years of medical practice, that muscle tension and pain is worse when women are under emotional stress. The more day-to-day stress that you have, related to family, work, and other personal issues, the more you may experience increased muscle tension and pain. Many of my patients have told me that their unhealed family and other personal relations, as well as sexual problems, are also significant emotional triggers for their sensations of pain and discomfort.

This exercise uses breathing to help you release any negative feelings, such as chronic anger or upset that you may be harboring. The more time you spend cleansing old negative emotional patterns, the less these feelings can create pain and tension in your body.

Lie flat on your back with your knees pulled up. Keep your feet slightly apart. Try to breathe in and out through your nose.

- Inhale deeply and see yourself enveloped in a soft white light. Breathe this light into every cell of your body. This is a cleansing light and can help wash away fear, anger, anxiety, and other negative feelings.

- As you exhale deeply, feel the light washing these emotions away.

- Repeat this exercise until you feel emotionally peaceful and clear.

Aerobic Exercise

Besides deep breathing exercises, I also recommend engaging in regular aerobic exercise like walking, swimming, dancing, bicycling and yoga. Aerobic exercise refers to any type of exercise that increases the amount of oxygen contained in the body.

With aerobic exercise, you receive the great benefit of combining deep, slow breathing with movement. Not only does it energize your body and elevate your mood, but aerobic exercise has great health benefits for your entire body including improving your resistance to respiratory infections!

When you engage in aerobic exercise, you create a pumping action of the muscles that helps to move oxygen, blood, and nutrients throughout the body. With regular aerobic exercise, skeletal muscles become energized and toned, making every movement—from lifting objects to walking—more easily accomplished.

This includes the muscles of the heart and lungs. As a result, aerobic exercise also conditions the heart and lungs to work more efficiently. As the heart becomes conditioned, it is able to pump more blood with each stroke. Thus, it can circulate the same volume of blood with fewer strokes and doesn't have to work as hard.

The lungs benefit, too, from aerobic exercise. Regular aerobic exercise helps us to breathe more deeply and efficiently, thereby improving oxygenation and nutrient flow to tissues throughout the entire body. With this type of exercise, you will tend to breathe more deeply and slowly. Over time, this helps to improve the elasticity of your lungs and relaxes the diaphragm and chest muscles, thereby allowing you to inhale more oxygen

It also aids in the removal of waste products such as carbon dioxide, lactic acid, and other products of metabolism through exhalation by the lungs. All of these benefits help to improve your resistance to respiratory infections.

I recommend that you engage in aerobic exercise like walking, swimming or bicycling at least 4 to 5 times per week. Doing some form of aerobic exercise every day for 30 to 60 minutes is even better! Walking is my favorite type of aerobic exercise. I am an avid walker, and have been since medical school—I walk at a moderate pace, breathing slowly and deeply to maximize the health and relaxation benefits. Often I walk with friends or family members. I have regular walking partners who I get together with and always look forward to talking and sharing with them as we walk together.

I live in the San Francisco Bay Area and there is a lot of natural beauty here- the bay, the surrounding mountains, lots of local parks, gardens and walking trails. We always try to find new places to explore. I love to walk after work, which helps to melt away the stress of my busy day. I also get to enjoy the beautiful natural surroundings of the area that I live in while receiving the fabulous health benefits of regular exercise, which is why I do it nearly every day.

The days I'm not able to get out, I can literally feel a subtle drop in my energy level, and my mood isn't as cheery and bright. Walking also helps to keep me flexible and has kept my weight virtually the same as when I was in medical school. My patients who are prone to respiratory infections have also found that they are much stronger, more energetic and develop colds, flus and bronchitis much less frequently.

In summary, my five step program to combat respiratory infections consists of 1) Destroying cold, flu, and lung infection causing microbes 2) Supporting healthy pH balance and alkalinity within your cells and tissues 3) Reducing inflammation through the use of digestive enzymes and other anti-inflammatory substances 4) Supporting healthy detoxification 5) Promoting healthy oxygenation

Given what a nuisance colds, flus, sinusitis, middle ear infections and bronchitis can be in terms of suffering from uncomfortable symptoms, a diminished quality of life, as well as loss of time on the job or engaging in enjoyable activities, I'm delighted that I have been able to share my program with you.

My program to combat and prevent respiratory infections has helped restore improved immunity and resistance to cold, flus and bronchitis to many of my patients and I hope that you find it to be very beneficial, as well.

About Susan Richards, M.D.

Dr. Susan Richards is one of the foremost authorities in the fields of family medicine and alternative medicine. Dr. Richards has successfully treated many thousands of patients emphasizing alternative health and integrative medicine in her clinical practice. Her mission is to provide her patients with safe and effective alternative therapies to greatly enhance their health and well-being.

A graduate of Northwestern University Feinberg School of Medicine, she has served on the clinical faculty of Stanford University School of Medicine and taught in their Division of Family and Community Medicine.

Her Facebook page, Dr. Susan's Healthy Living, has over one million followers. She is also an ordained minister and her ministry receives over a million prayer requests for healing each year.

NOTES

NOTES

NOTES

www.ingramcontent.com/pod-product-compliance
Lightning Source LLC
Chambersburg PA
CBHW070907290526
45795CB00001B/241